The Lord
The Lover
The Life Coach

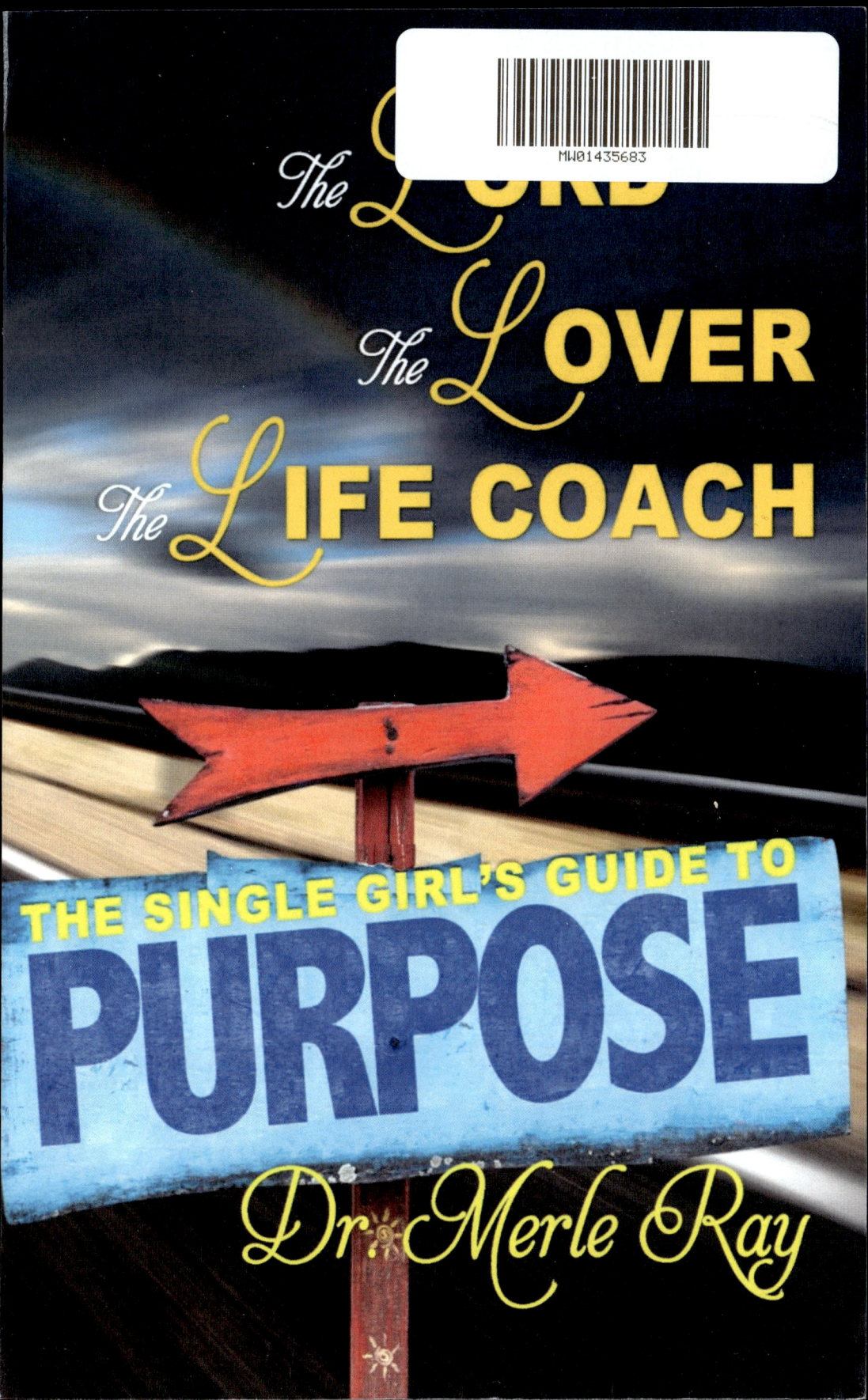

The Single Girl's Guide to PURPOSE

Dr. Merle Ray

DIVINE SEED

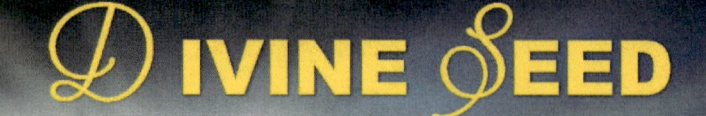

AN OVERVIEW AND EXPLORATION TOOL

Thirty minutes. That's how long it took me to conceive. But it took me nearly 30 years to believe what I received.

When the Spirit of God touched my heart, I was driving home from work. Listening to love songs by Bebe and CeCe Winans, God, the Lover said to me, *"I wish you would let me love on you like that!"*

Dr. Merle Ray,

The Brilliance Coach©

Business & Life Strategist

The Lord. The Lover. The Life Coach.
SERIES™

The Single Girl's Guide to Purpose™
By Dr. Merle Ray
Pregnant on Purpose™
30-minutes to Divine Seed – An Overview and Exploration Tool

Published by The Noble Groups on the Amazon Independent Platform
Printed in the U.S.A.

ISBN: 9798590683543

Contact: mhray@DrMerleRay.com
Web: www.DrMerleRay.com
Web: www.RealWomanhood.com

All rights reserved. No part of this book may be reproduced or transmitted in any form or by any means, electronic or mechanical, including photocopy, recording, or by any information storage and retrieval system, without written permission from the author, except for the inclusion of brief quotations in a review.

Copyright © 2020 by Dr. Merle Ray.
All Rights Reserved.

REALWomanhood: The Business and Calling of Being a Woman is the intellectual property of Dr. Merle Ray. Logo is intended to be a trademark registered in the United States Patent and Trademark Office by The Noble Groups. Use of either in any form requires written permission from the author.

Unless otherwise indicated, Bible quotations are taken from The Holy Bible King James Version, Public Domain.

This book is not to be construed as legal, medical, technical, business, professional or personally devised spiritual counseling or advise. See Disclaimer at back of book.

The Lord. The Lover. The Life Coach.
SERIES™

DISCLAIMER:

I would like to make it understood that I am in no way associated with the medical, psychological, or physiological profession. I do not offer the information included in this book as a substitute for professional advice, mental health or medical treatment. This book is for general knowledge and reading pleasure only. I offer no results and also do not take responsibility for any individual's mental, physical, or spiritual health, well-being or illness; nor am I responsible for their healing. I offer no guarantee that anyone will have results by reading this book or receive a life that is filled with their desire, dream, or vision for themselves, or a life that is stress free, or that any physical, social, spiritual, emotional or mental disorder, disease, or illness will be prevented.

I do, however, believe that we are spirit beings who have a soul and live in a body according to I Thessalonians 5:23. I also believe that most problems that manifest in the behavior, soul, and body of a woman have a spiritual root. And I believe that Jesus paid the price for our physical, spiritual, and mental well-being (Isaiah 53:5, I Peter 2:24).

It is not my intent to lay any other foundation for the Gospel than that founded by Jesus Christ, My Lord. With this, I do believe that women have a wider definition and purpose from God than what we've been shown in our various cultures and environments. God is the One who created us and destined us for greatness from the very beginning. In that, I believe God is the same yesterday, today, and forever more – we are built for greatness!

My goal is not to debate religion or complain about church people in this book, for I am a Believer in Christ. I love My Father God and my debate is not with Him or Christ's church! My call is to expose the lies of the world, the lies of our culture, and the lies of the enemy that I once believed – and to replace them with the love and truth of God's Word as my new set of beliefs.

Further, nothing in this book is offered as professional advice or expertise. Please do not take anything in this book as legal, technical, medical, business, personal, health, relationships, or other advice. The words offered are my beliefs, my story only offered in encouragement to you to find your story and your beliefs in the Word of God. I encourage you to seek out your own solutions, when needed, working with your own team of specialized experts in their fields for any issue plaguing your life, and may God bless you.

The Lord. The Lover. The Life Coach.
SERIES™

THE SINGLE GIRL'S GUIDE TO PURPOSE

Pregnant on Purpose™

30-minutes to Divine Seed

An Overview and Exploration Tool

Introduction 7
    Pregnant On Purpose................................... 9
    Ready to Love 29
The Pregnant Man.. 39
Don't Sleep With My Husband............................ 70
    My Partner of Purpose 70
Day 1 – Knowing What You Believe 78
Day 2 – Checking Your Heart.............................. 81
Day 3 – Entreating The Lord............................... 91
Day 4 – Removing the 'Ungreat'........................ 95
Day 5 – Letting God Dance Over You 99
    Healing My Libido 99
Day 6 – Knowing the Full Package..................... 103
    Intimacy, Beauty, and Adventure 103
Day 7 – Planning for the Best Dates Ever!........ 108

Pregnant on Purpose

The Lord. The Lover. The Life **Coach.**
SERIES™

IMPORTANT

This BOOK is an Overview and Exploration tool which serves as a Workbook, Diary, or Journal of coaching exercises to increase your spiritual growth and effectiveness in becoming spiritually pregnant. The paperback version is suggested to write and capture your thoughts in during the pondering questions and exploration in order to get the most use out of the book. Topics: Intimacy with God, dating and intimacy with purpose partners, growing in your potential for personal, professional, and spiritual productivity, and sacred intimacy based on Scripture.

eBook and Paperback versions available on Amazon.com.

Pregnant on Purpose

Introduction

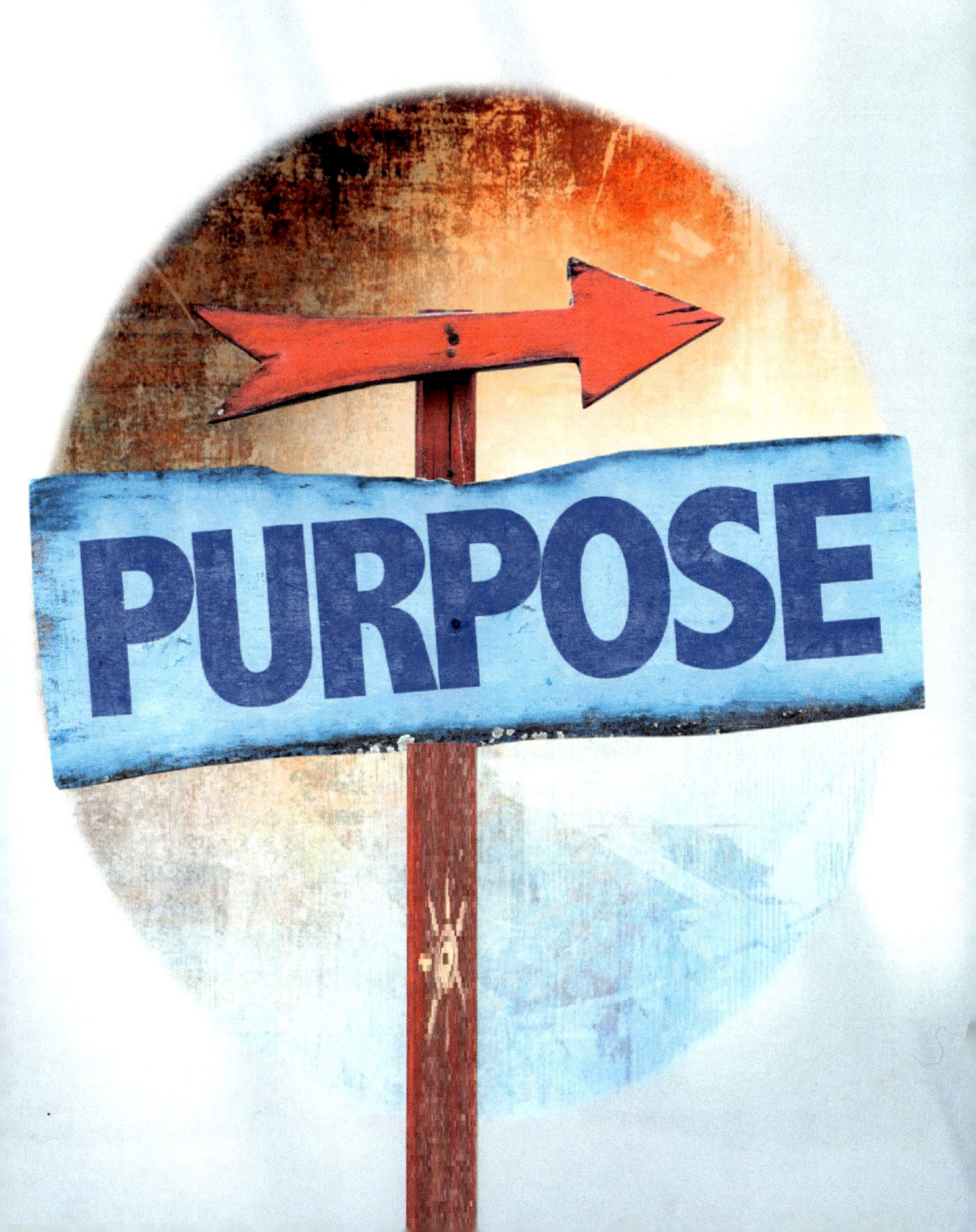

The Lord. The Lover. The Life Coach.
SERIES™

Thirty minutes. That's how long it took me to conceive. But it took me nearly 30 years to believe what I received.

When the Spirit of God spoke to my heart, I was driving home from work. Listening to love songs by Bebe and CeCe Winans, God, the Lover said to me,

> "I wish you would let me love on you like that!"

After the foreplay was over, and a metaphorical nine months of carrying REAL seed, there it was – God's brilliant birthing and my breakthrough to greater!

GREATER LIFE. GREATER LOVE.
GREATER ADVENTURE.

Pregnant on Purpose

The Lord. The Lover. The Life Coach.
SERIES™

Pregnant on Purpose

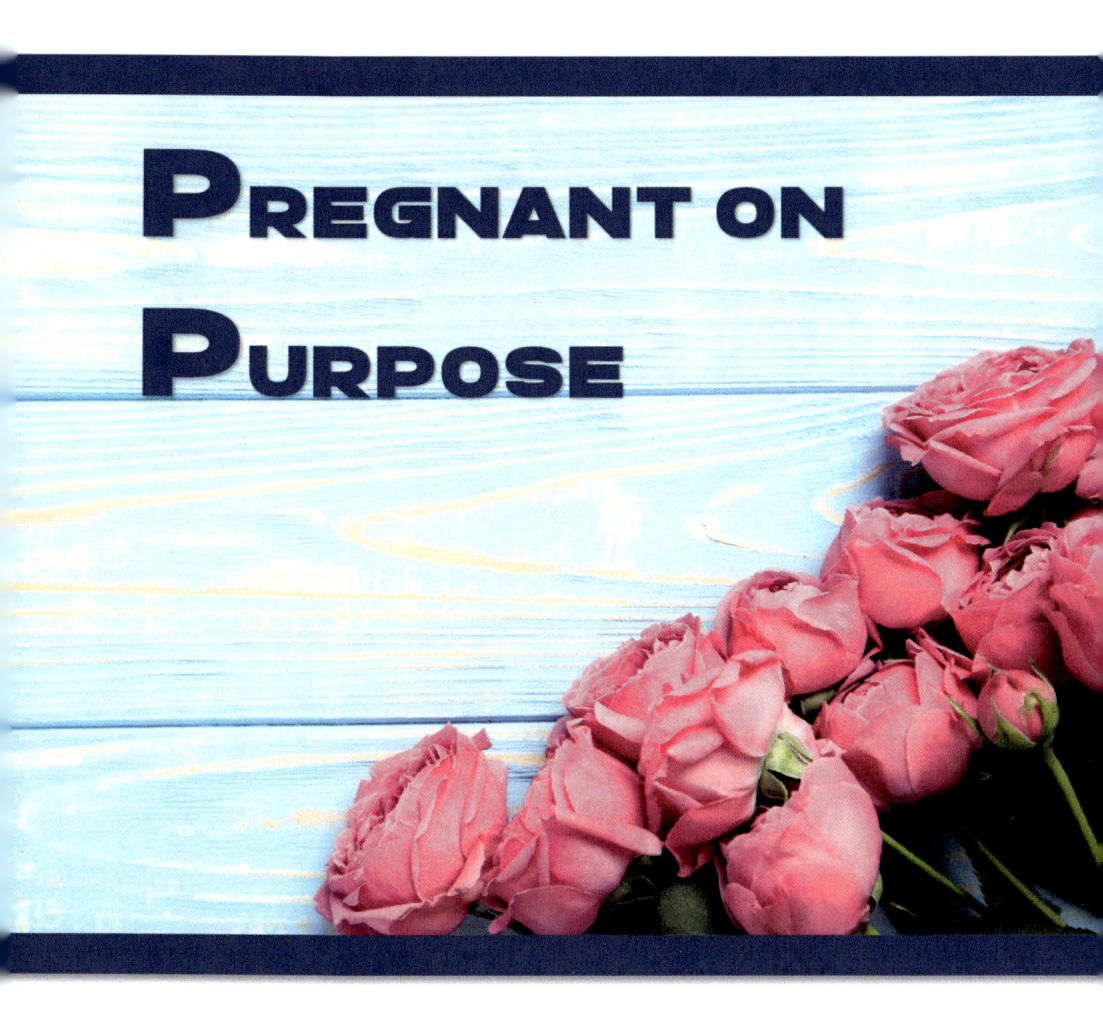

Especially for adult women AND the men that love them, this book is an overview and exploration tool, a coaching workbook designed to guide you through concepts that I have used to become spiritually

Pregnant on Purpose

The Lord. The Lover. The Life Coach.
SERIES™

pregnant and to conceive every single time – getting pregnant on purpose!

Whether you are wanting to birth: a baby, a relationship, a business, or a book, God doesn't give accidental blessings. His blessings are all about PURPOSE.

During this time of unprecedented trial, challenge, and change, there's still no better time than the present to conceive God's brilliant plan and purpose for your life!

Single individuals and married couples will want to explore each exercise in this workbook! Watch what happens as you yield yourself to God!

The Lord. The Lover. The Life Coach.
SERIES™

God doesn't give accidental blessings.

His blessings are all about PURPOSE.

Pregnant on Purpose

The Lord. The Lover. The Life Coach.
SERIES™

Are You Pregnant?
Trying to Get Pregnant?
At-risk?
Or About to Deliver?

At a time when many couples are not trying to get pregnant, why would God be speaking about becoming **Pregnant on Purpose**?

Look around you. How many love-starved people do you see?

Men and women are still looking for love, especially now. When COVID-19 was publicized, online dating increased and caught aflame like wildfire. It has more than tripled on dating apps like Tinder, Plenty of Fish, and Bumble reporting increases of 30% to 119%[i]. Social media sites like Facebook have added dating apps and experts have already predicted that the world is in for another baby boom which is due in about four to six more months from the time of this entry into the book (July-September 2020) which would be about nine to twelve months since March 2020, the announcement of the devastating global pandemic hitting the United States.

At 57 years old, upon hearing of people dropping off the face of the planet like flies, I began to ask myself, is this the way it is going to be? I've always known that more difficult times were coming as the time draws near for Christ to return, but somehow I guess I thought things would be different. I thought I'd have accomplished all that was in my heart to accomplish with God on this side of the sun. I began to look at my life and wonder what was missing. God has been good to me and I have no complaints, but the one thing that was missing in my life now, was a physical sacred romance. I truly felt that I'd not had the beauty, intimacy, and adventure that I sought in a loving relationship with a man.

As times became more desperate, businesses closing, unemployment off the charts everywhere, stock market tumbling in decline, food and household items scarcely on the grocery store shelves, airplanes nearly empty, and more and more people dying, I had only one desire. I wanted to make love. Not have sex, I wanted to love and be loved by a man on earth who loved me uninhibitedly, undeniably, and untarnished. I did not want to leave this earth not having known what that was like. Was this even possible now? I've been divorced several times. The whole world is in a standstill and practicing for the first time ever in my generation – a term that I'd never heard before – social distancing. Standing 6 feet apart from each other, with the whole world on lockdown, how was I going to receive the blessing now? The blessing was to love and be loved by a man!

Once again, I had to enter into the bed chambers of God. This time, unlike before, I knew who I was. When I started writing my first book nearly 15 years ago, I didn't know who I was. But this time, I had my Spiritual Identity intact. I knew who I was, whose I was, and what is my destiny. This time, I just wanted to be loved on this side of the sun by another human being, a male counterpart – a man.

It had been some time since I was this serious about being in a relationship. Why was the thought of being in a relationship with a man coming back up now? I was feeling somewhat alienated from the rest of the world who had companionship. I didn't know if it was because of the pandemic, feelings of uncertainty, and the sheer fright of losing so many people in the world at once or what. All I knew however was that I had to go back into God's secret chambers and find out from Him what was going on within me.

I was panicking. Upon the news that the world was in a state of global pandemic and becoming fearful, seeing people that I knew and loved affected who now were gone, and thousands upon thousands more being added to the numbers week after week, I was feeling alone and afraid.

I wasn't as afraid that the end time might be near. I was more afraid that I hadn't lived out all of who God had called me to be on earth while I was here. I was thinking of every promise I had still in my heart to live out, like the promise of being made a happy wife. That wasn't the only promise I wanted to live out. But I began to realize how much I hadn't yet lived out my full potential. I quickly understood that my longing wasn't just about being in a fulfilled relationship, but being more fully engaged with God in my purpose especially in

The Lord. The Lover. The Life Coach. SERIES™

such a tumultuous time on earth – **becoming pregnant on purpose!**

Is it possible to love God and be intimate with Him today during worldwide crisis in such a way as to be filled with His Glory, become pregnant, conceive and deliver his full promises even though the world is in chaos? What about when the delivery that you are believing God for is a healthy thriving relationship with a person of the opposite sex? Doesn't that seem a bit shallow given a global pandemic and the dire situations that we are in today?

> *"When I was growing up we had a word for women and girls who used to get pregnant on purpose."*

How many times have you seen and heard of women who were in relationships that they feared would be lost? What did they do to keep the guys around? They would get pregnant on purpose! To be honest, I wanted to get pregnant on purpose at

The Lord. The Lover. The Life Coach.
SERIES™

first just to get God's attention – to keep things the way they were before the pandemic. Honestly, I was wishing that He would push this pandemic thing far away from us with good riddance! At 57 years old, I certainly was not thinking about a physical pregnancy. Now, because of the situation the world is in, I was rushing to grasp hold of all the remaining dreams, goals, and promises that I have from God, not knowing how much time we have left on this side of the sun. I was wanting to become **pregnant on purpose**!

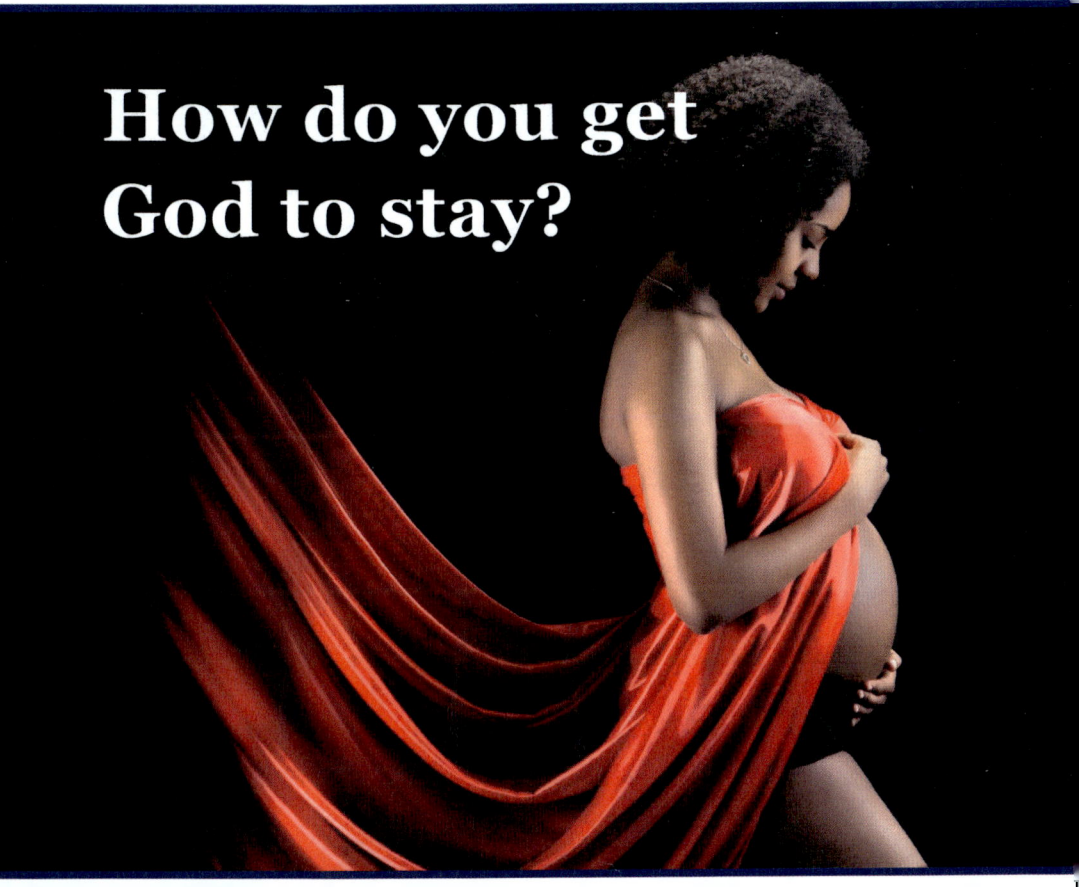

How do you get God to stay?

The Lord. The Lover. The Life Coach. SERIES™

Single Girl's Dilemma

How do you get God's attention when it seems that He is busy doing much more important work on earth?

With the world around us seeming to prophetically line up to come to a head, we don't know how long we have left on this side of the sun. This is – the only side where we can be in a relationship of the opposite sex with a person ordained by God to have dominion. So, how can we still enjoy and fulfill His purpose on earth? God has given us the ability to have physical and spiritual babies here,

Pregnant on Purpose

The Lord. The Lover. The Life Coach.
SERIES™

and share dominion with our earthly co-partners and counterparts on this side of the sun. On the other side, there will be no need for such relationships because there is no marriage or giving in marriage relationships in heaven.

In heaven, human beings will no longer be single or married as we will be in a totally different bodily state. We'll all be at home in our new bodies as one with God. Make no mistake about it: we may be at or near the end of this present world as we know it; but be of good cheer, we are being prepared for a different world where we are in the presence of God all the time fully satisfied content and at peace where time, distress, lack and tears are irrelevant.

So how do we who love God and want to experience His fulfillment on this side of the sun right now do that? With the time we have left here how do we continue to pursue our destiny, purpose, and dreams when so much is going on that we have no control over? How do those who wish to be in healthy happy thriving relationships do so in this world with so many changes affecting our daily lives? What about those who want to make a difference in the world through business,

The Lord. The Lover. The Life Coach.
SERIES™

or those who wish to impact lives around the world? And what about the single moms who have children already – physical children? They want to raise productive successful children as citizens of this generation. How do they do that now with all that's going on around us? How can the single mom prepare her children for what's coming in this generation and the next? We don't know the answers to all of what's coming, but what we do know is that we – as single women and moms have to get ourselves together first before we can be and do what we're called to be and do. I call that – **REAL Womanhood: The Business and Calling of Being a Woman**[ii]. Our families, our children, and those who look to us for civility, stability, and so much more deserve to know that we're going to be able to stand during these times no matter what happens. When the world is in so much turmoil and uncertainty, where is the single girl's blessed assurance of God's presence, power, pardon, promise, provision, and prosperity while we yet live on earth?

Pregnant on Purpose

The Lord. The Lover. The Life Coach.
SERIES™

How do we become spiritually pregnant and conceive God's brilliant plan, purpose, and promises for our lives during a time of unprecedented trial, challenge, and change in the earth?

Psalm 65:4
Blessed is the woman whom thou choosest, and causest to approach unto thee, that she may dwell in thy courts: we shall be satisfied with the goodness of thy house, even of thy holy temple.

Pregnant on Purpose

FROM THE AUTHOR

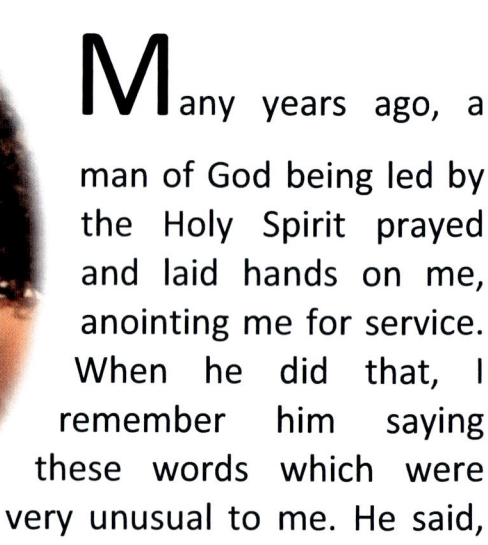

Many years ago, a man of God being led by the Holy Spirit prayed and laid hands on me, anointing me for service. When he did that, I remember him saying these words which were very unusual to me. He said, *"That which would have been unlawful."*

At the time when the man of God said those words over me, I did not know what they meant. As God began to deal with me over time, I began to notice a pattern. Whenever God would visit me, I would gain revelation of His Word, and God would give me understanding in very intimate ways. Many times, the Holy Spirit would use romantic terminology

Pregnant on Purpose

and that would peak my interest. I began to desire God's presence around me more. I used to have the desire to be filled and loved by a man. So every time I sought God, He would always show me an example of what He was saying in physical terms of love and intimacy. I believe it is because that's what I always wanted most in my life, to be loved by a man who would cherish me as Christ loves the church. So when I received the title for this book, **Pregnant on Purpose**, I was not surprised.

That's how God, my Love, has spoken to me since I was about 30. My conversations, presentations, and journeys have always somehow led me to center on Christ and a particular focus of His will in a person, place, or thing, as it relates to being loved and having intimacy with God.

What is real love and affection? What it is, and what it is not, I believe, is the basis for all things on earth. From governments to industries to education – heck, even with our jobs. We will either love them or hate them. We either have passion for what it is that we do for a living, or we don't. The same holds true for everything in life!

Everyone who creates something, or builds a business, or teaches a child, or raises family, or

The Lord. The Lover. The Life Coach.
SERIES™

runs for political office, either loves himself and what he is doing or not. So to me, love is the basis for all things.

Think about it. If we had love, we wouldn't need the police. Don't you dare talk about defunding the police when there isn't enough love in the world. We need the law on this side of the sun because we do not have enough love. We would not need to have a greener environment if we had love. We wouldn't even need as many hospitals or doctors if love was our foundation. There are numerous types of love, and the three types that I am referring to most often in this book are romantic love (eros), enduring love (pragma), and playful love (ludis) because most often these three are prevalent in relationships leading to romance and marriage.

God has never approached me in the usual religious ways; He has always been very personal. When I have had encounters with Him, they have always been intimate on His part, and I have always left pregnant – that is, with His seed growing inside of me.

Such is the case with this book. I'm believing God that will be the case with you too. Prepare to

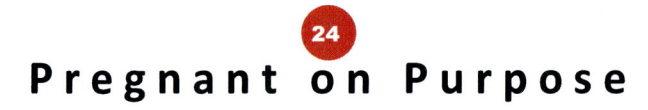

Pregnant on Purpose

The Lord. The Lover. The Life Coach.
SERIES™

become pregnant on purpose and birth the brilliant plan God has for your life using His principles. Don't presume you already know about these topics as you read this book; you don't how God is planning on bringing the blessing to pass. Just be open to His leading as you read each short segment, and then complete the exploration questions included for you to ponder as you apply what you receive in this workbook.

Of course, we recognize that it's not just single women who are affected by the trials, challenges, and turbulence in the world right now. Married women and girls everywhere are included within the central themes of this book. Even men will benefit from taking a thought-provoking look at the inner-man using the pondering questions and banner messages scattered throughout this book. If for no other reason than to understand and support the plight of their moms, wives, daughters, sisters, nieces, associates, friends and loved ones, men who desire to read this book and apply godly wisdom and love in the care of the women connected to them are tremendously appreciated, blessed, and we pray, rewarded by our Father, God.

Pregnant on Purpose

The Lord. The Lover. The Life **Coach.**
SERIES™

Greater understanding, greater revelation, enlightenment, and clarity will become yours as you move in the direction of seeking God for yourself through these insightful topics. This is what happened for me, and I believe that every person listening and reading is included. YOU too can become spiritually pregnant, and birth God's brilliant plan for your life!

Presumptions/Assumptions

Take a moment to reflect how you thought the blessing(s) was going to come in your life. *What have you assumed about God? Your blessings? Purpose? What do you believe to be true today?*

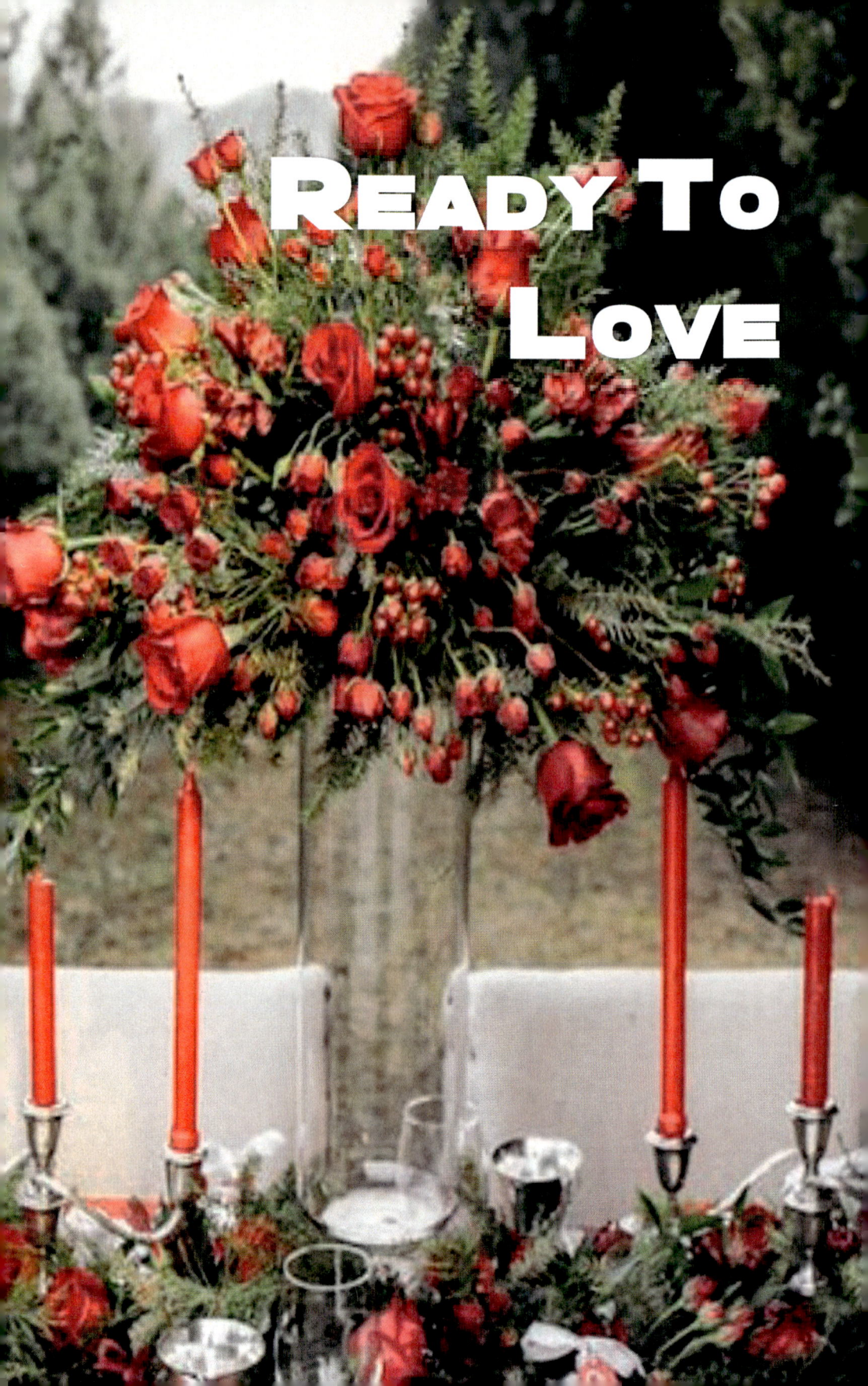

Ready To Love

The Lord. The Lover. The Life Coach.
SERIES™

READY TO LOVE

In previous books, I have walked you through journeys in which God and I have shared intimate encounters and always as a result, after that, the promises of God have been birthed in my life. In my first book, **Spiritual Identity**, I shared how to fall in love with God and find out who you are in the process. In **Six Figures and Beyond Success**, I have shared how intimacy with God can birth business and career changes in your life to propel you to the next level. In **Meantime** and **40-days to Transformation**, I have shared how God nurtures you, picks you up and transforms your life when your spiritual fathers, mothers, or others who you respect and admire seem to drop you, and when life in general seems to become too tough to manage.

Today in this book I'll show you how the Lord can take you from singleness of heart with Him to bring you to a point of readiness to share your life with the world and others in healthy ways no matter what's going on around you. I'll show you how to become Pregnant

Pregnant on Purpose

The Lord. The Lover. The Life Coach.
SERIES™

on purpose with God's seed and share it with someone you love. Many of us want a loving relationship, but we are empty inside, and do not know how to love ourselves. However, we want someone who loves God and who would cherish us. Yet, we do not know how to set our faith to be open to receive God's seed being in love with Him first. Believe me, if there is a mate in this world for you, it is for God's purpose. Truly, I believe that it does not take God forever to move. Instead, I believe that God is indeed waiting on us to move!

How you move is important. The promise of things we are hoping for from God is waiting on our substance. By substance, I mean our faith in Him, which is belief and readiness. In other words, our preparation for the blessing is essential. The longer I live, the more I have realized in life that the blessing has always come, but sometimes I have not recognized the blessing when it came, or I was not successful in handling the blessing because I was unprepared when the blessing came.

Zig Ziglar, a phenomenal business entrepreneur, motivational speaker and well-known former salesperson used to say, *"Success is when preparation meets opportunity."* When I

The Lord. The Lover. The Life Coach. SERIES™

heard that, it occurred to me that **Preparation** is just another word for obedience. If you think about it, as believers, God sends us instructions and it seems like the moment our minds lay hold on the word, "obedience," we consciously or subconsciously shut down. But today, the Holy Spirit impressed upon me that I should not automatically shirk when I hear the word "obedience."

We church people automatically think of obedience as hard. But business people don't; they prepare all the time. In fact, everyday working professionals, top performers, and business people embrace the concept of preparation and they are rewarded for it. Preparation, when it is being realized or put out is simply cultivation, another word for work. That's why God says in His word, *"Faith without works is dead."* God doesn't want us to work for the blessing, but He does want us to prepare for it! He's giving us the blessing, so we don't have to work for it. No, it's a blessing and a gift from God by nature is something good for us, not bad *(Jeremiah 29:11)*.

> **God doesn't want us to work for the blessing, but He does want us to prepare for it!**

The Lord. The Lover. The Life Coach.
SERIES™

We're also going to receive the gift from God because the Bible says, *"the gifts of God are without repentance."* That means, the blessings will come, regardless of whether we deserve the gifts or not. God does not take away the gifts, and we will not have to work for them.

But here's the thing: **faith without works is dead**, God's Word says in James chapter 2. What? Bummer! Doesn't that sound like God is reneging? I know, right? But get this. There's a reason why faith without works is dead, and it's not because God needs any work from us.

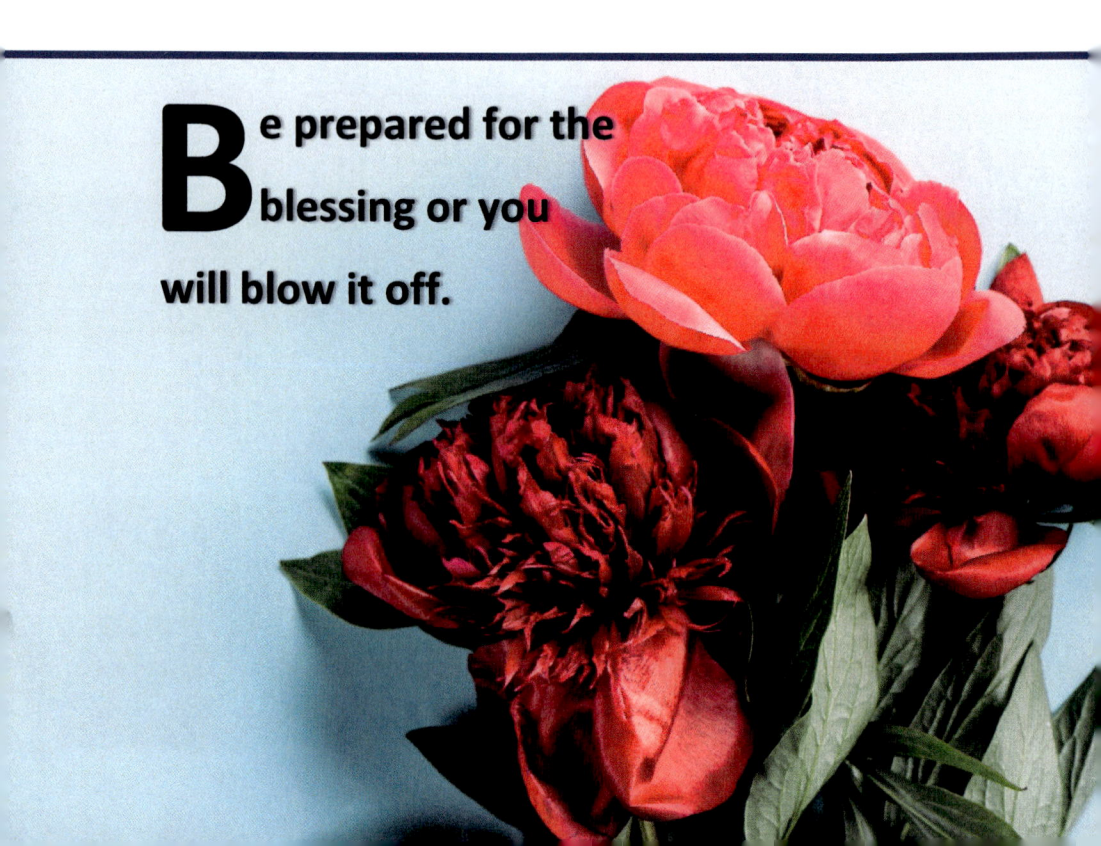

Be prepared for the blessing or you will blow it off.

The Lord. The Lover. The Life Coach.
SERIES™

Transformation is possible for you. Thus, the reason for this book. Many of us are thinking, – 'I must have already blown it off because it certainly hasn't happened for me yet.' Without realizing it, the truth is the blessing may have already come, but we were so poorly prepared that we didn't recognize it! We love to say that God is in control, and the truth is, yes. God is in control in that He's sovereign over heaven and earth. Everything belongs to Him, and will ultimately bow down to His presence over all things. However, God doesn't stop or overrule man's dominion on earth. He has given you dominion to make choices while you are on this earth.

If God was going to control every move you made as a person, don't you think He would have controlled Eve's choices in the garden? The truth is God gave man dominion over man's choices. And you have a lot more control over your destiny than you think. Does this mean that you've blown every chance you have for happiness? No, because every day is a new gift from God!

With so much going on in the world today, we may feel that it's too late for anything good. Is it too late for us to fall in love and enjoy a healthy

The Lord. The Lover. The Life Coach. SERIES™

thriving relationship? Are you thinking it's too late to be joyful or happy about life with someone of the opposite sex? We have our guards up. We're not trying to be in a relationship. It's just way too much trouble.

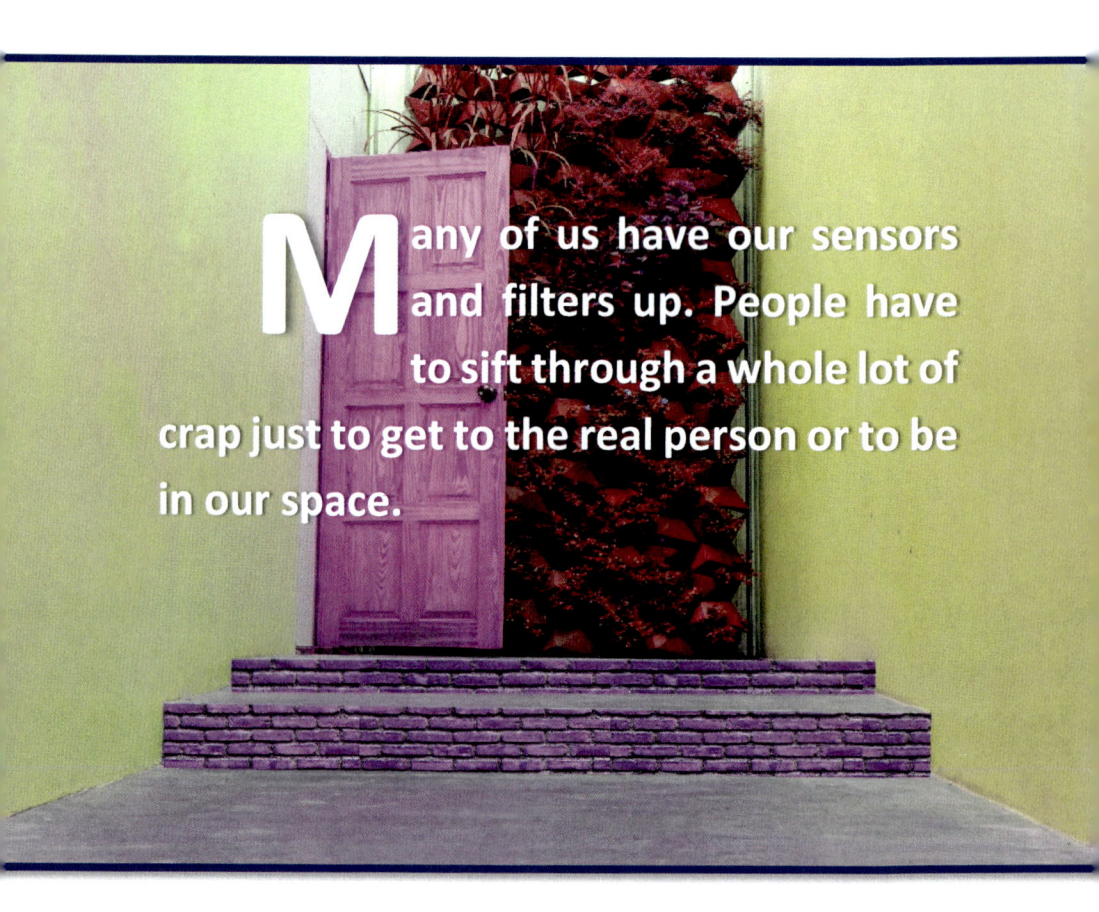

Many of us have our sensors and filters up. People have to sift through a whole lot of crap just to get to the real person or to be in our space.

Pregnant on Purpose

The Lord. The Lover. The Life Coach.
SERIES™

Others of us have been on dating sites for years without finding a mate. It seems impossible to meet someone of the opposite sex that we can talk to and understand. We are wondering what's wrong with us. You are saying, **"Why can't I find someone to love on and to love me back."** This statement is truly spoken by both women and men. Let's face it. We love God, but some of us – we are lonely.

Many of us are looking for relationships for the wrong reasons. We are looking to be in a relationship with another person only for what we can get out of it, not for what we have to give. This is not the kind of relationship that would thrive and grow and mutually bless each other. Love is not about taking but about giving, and by giving I do not merely mean material things, sex, or money. Love is about much more than the external.

If you can only give externally and do not know anything about how to give to a person internally, then God wants to visit with you today. If you want to be ready to love and don't know how, I believe all of that changes today as you give yourself to God. I pray that the principles and concepts shared in this book will help you. If you

Pregnant on Purpose

The Lord. The Lover. The Life Coach. SERIES™

are already a Believer, but you are frustrated and distraught because you feel that your life is still waiting to happen, then my prayer is that you will explore further the purpose God has for you.

An Exploration Tool

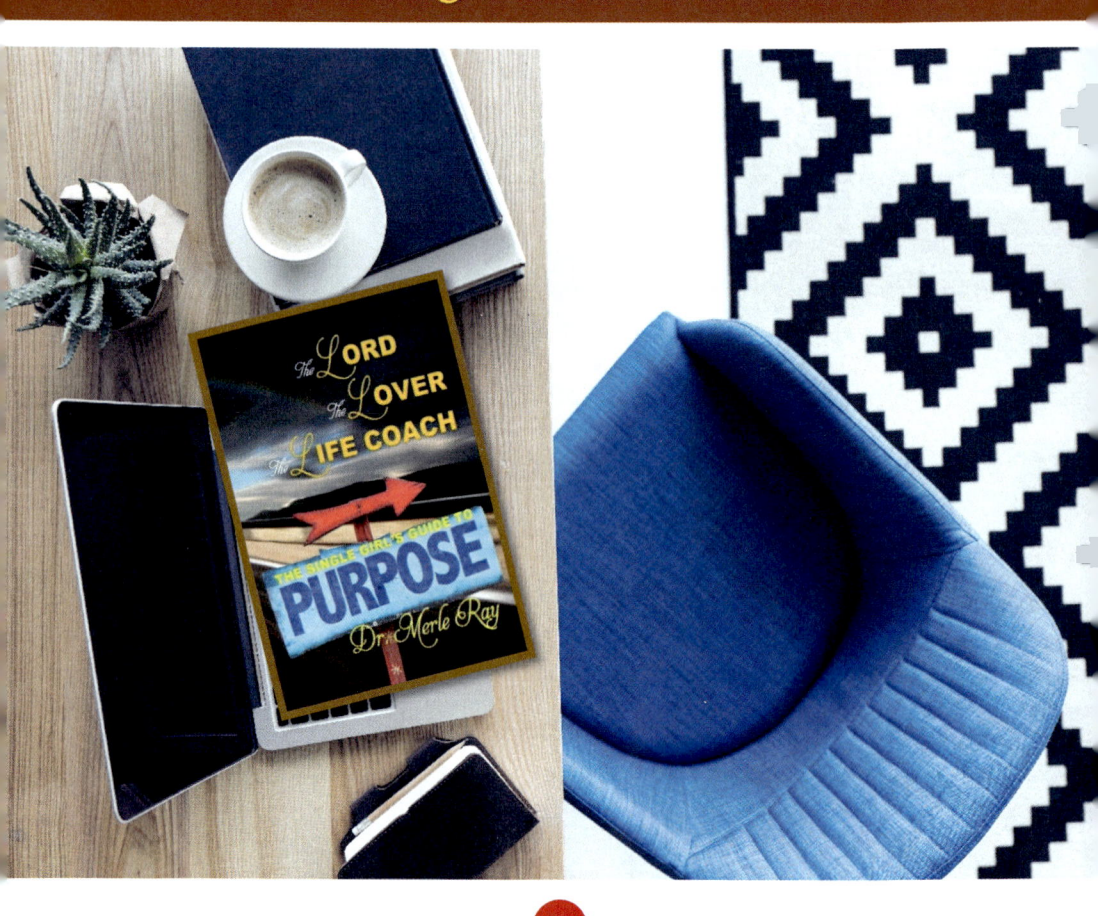

Pregnant on Purpose

Reflections

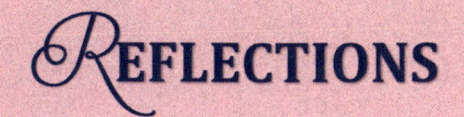

What methods have you tried in the past to become spiritually pregnant?

When have you tried to share your seed – your dreams, visions, and aspirations that God gave you to someone of the opposite sex?

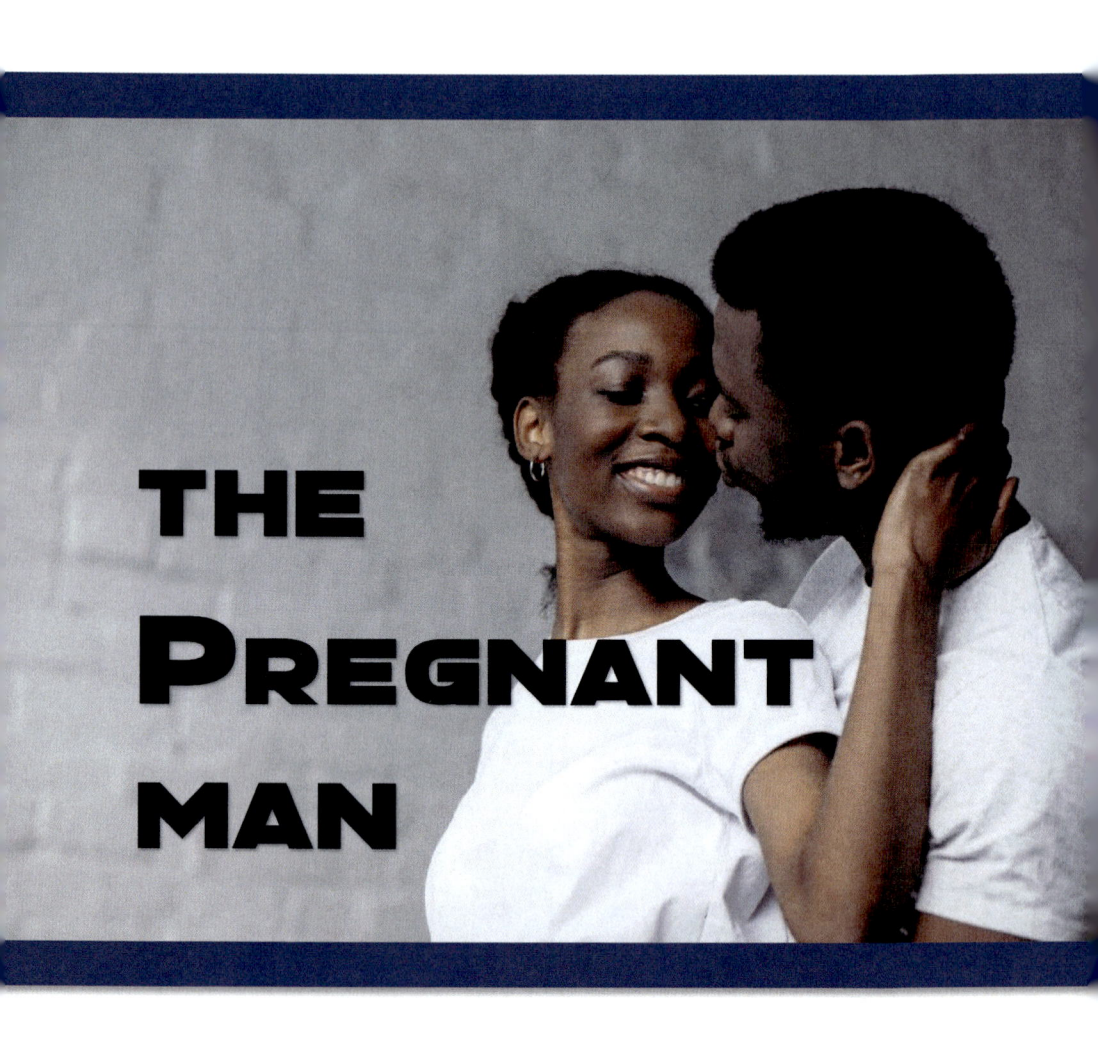

THE PREGNANT MAN

Pregnant on Purpose

The Lord. The Lover. The Life **Coach.**
SERIES™

THE PREGNANT MAN

In Genesis 3, God said to man, *"from dust you were taken and from dust you will return,"* and as I reflected on this Scripture the Lord said to me, *"Before you were dirt, you were my desire,"* and I realized that's how I got here. God desired to have a relationship with me. God wants to have a relationship with you. With God, we are not objects! We are relationships waiting to happen.

God had a world full of objects already, but He wanted relationships. Then He created mankind. I realized that like God, man desires wholesome fulfilled satisfying loving relationships too. That's where the desire comes from.

Pregnant on Purpose

The Lord. The Lover. The Life Coach.
SERIES™

Desire was designed to be filled with truth, not myths and lies. That's why desire is a good thing when it's filled by the spirit of God, and not by our lusts. The best way to fill the craving that a man has is to be filled in a thriving transparent free and open relationship with the deepness of who God is. The love of God makes a man fall to his knees. When God is the object of a man's affections, He arrests a man's intention so that a man does not destroy himself. God gives a man his own thoughts so that he can never get bored with conquering life. He fills a man's life with the pursuit of pleasure and purpose together. A man's responsibility is to become mature towards godly character, morale courage, and personal integrity, not to become attracted to pointless pains and meaningless pressures of life. How does God fill a man's life you ask?

God puts part of Himself into a man. When a man does not tap into the God-side of himself, he can feel worthless and devalued. God made you for something greater. When one refuses to see that, what good is he? The salt has lost its savor.

When a man believes in, trusts in, and gives in to the one and only Most Holy God, when he

Pregnant on Purpose

The Lord. The Lover. The Life Coach.
SERIES™

truly leans in to all of who God is to him, who God is in his life, his world, his hopes and dreams, then that man is established in himself and in the God that he yields himself to. This is why so many men are disappointed today in general with life, with women, with work, and with the world. A man is disappointed because of what or whom he has given himself over to.

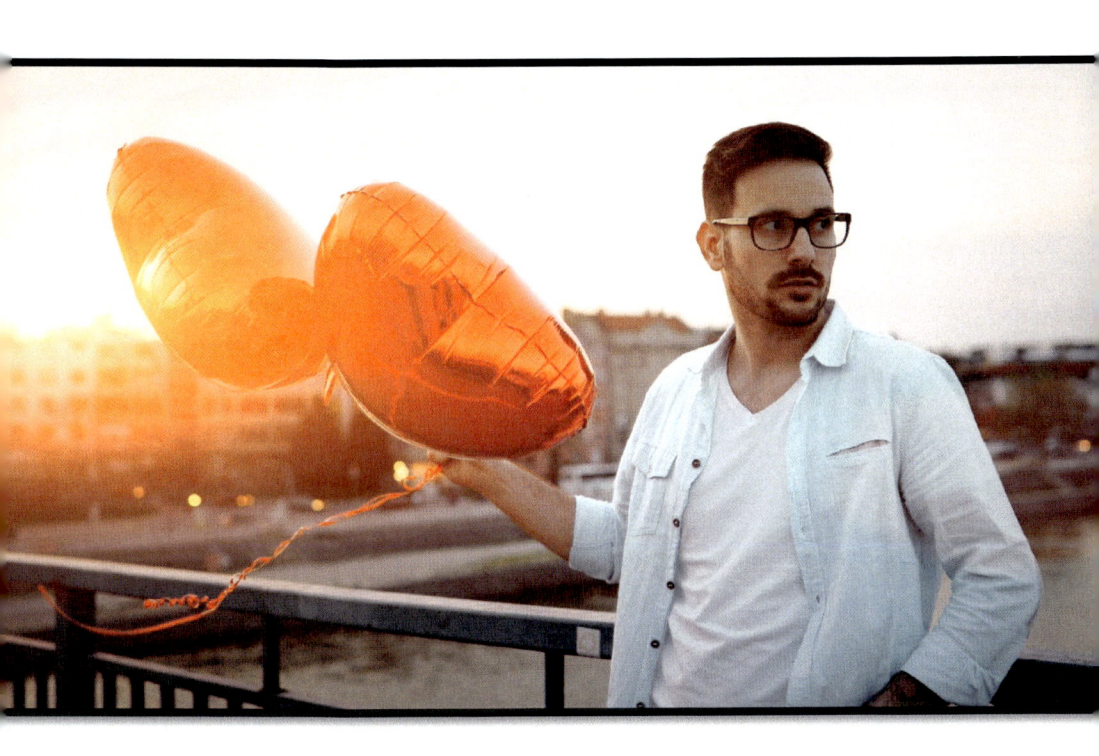

Pregnant on Purpose

The Lord. The Lover. The Life Coach.
SERIES™

A man needs to give himself, yield, fall down before in reverence to, and worship God because God is a part of him, and a man cannot ever be fully made whole or satisfied without God. Why? Because in God is where all the adventure a man seeks, the beauty he's captivated by, and the intimacy a man hopes for is found. It all comes from God. It may come through a woman, or work, or sports, but a man's healthy desires all stem from a holy place, God.

> **Man is never fulfilled without the essence of his spirit. The spirit man is the closest he'll ever be to God.**

Pregnant on Purpose

The Lord. The Lover. The Life Coach. SERIES™

God is in a man's character. God is in a man's toughness. God is in a man's loving kindness toward another human being. God is the secret that holds a man together throughout all his weaknesses, and God is the only one who can fill any void that a man has. God is intentional love! He will use anything and anyone that he wishes in order to make a man whole. But God does this by his own rules. God plays by his own game, and man doesn't even know the way to win God's heart. Yet, it's possible to please God. Not with our works, but with our **thoughts** towards Him, we can win God's heart. That's how we please Him – how we think about Him. God said to Job's friends, you have not done as my servant, Job, and thought of me.

This book will help you **think of Him**. If you want to receive the blessing of God, then shouldn't your thoughts be of Him? Take note, God is a romantic! He likes to be courted. He wants to be known and understood for who He really is, but the problem is no one wants to know. We think we know already. But we are missing out on one big love story because the

Pregnant on Purpose

secret of being in love with another human being is knowing God. Get in the practice of seeking Him like a Lover. You will find that He really is. Then, you'll better understand the true meaning of love!

Reflections

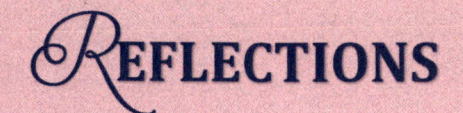

Who are other pregnant people in your life at the moment?

How do you spend quality time with others with whom you can share dreams, goals, visions, aspirations? How relevant are they for the gift that you are carrying?

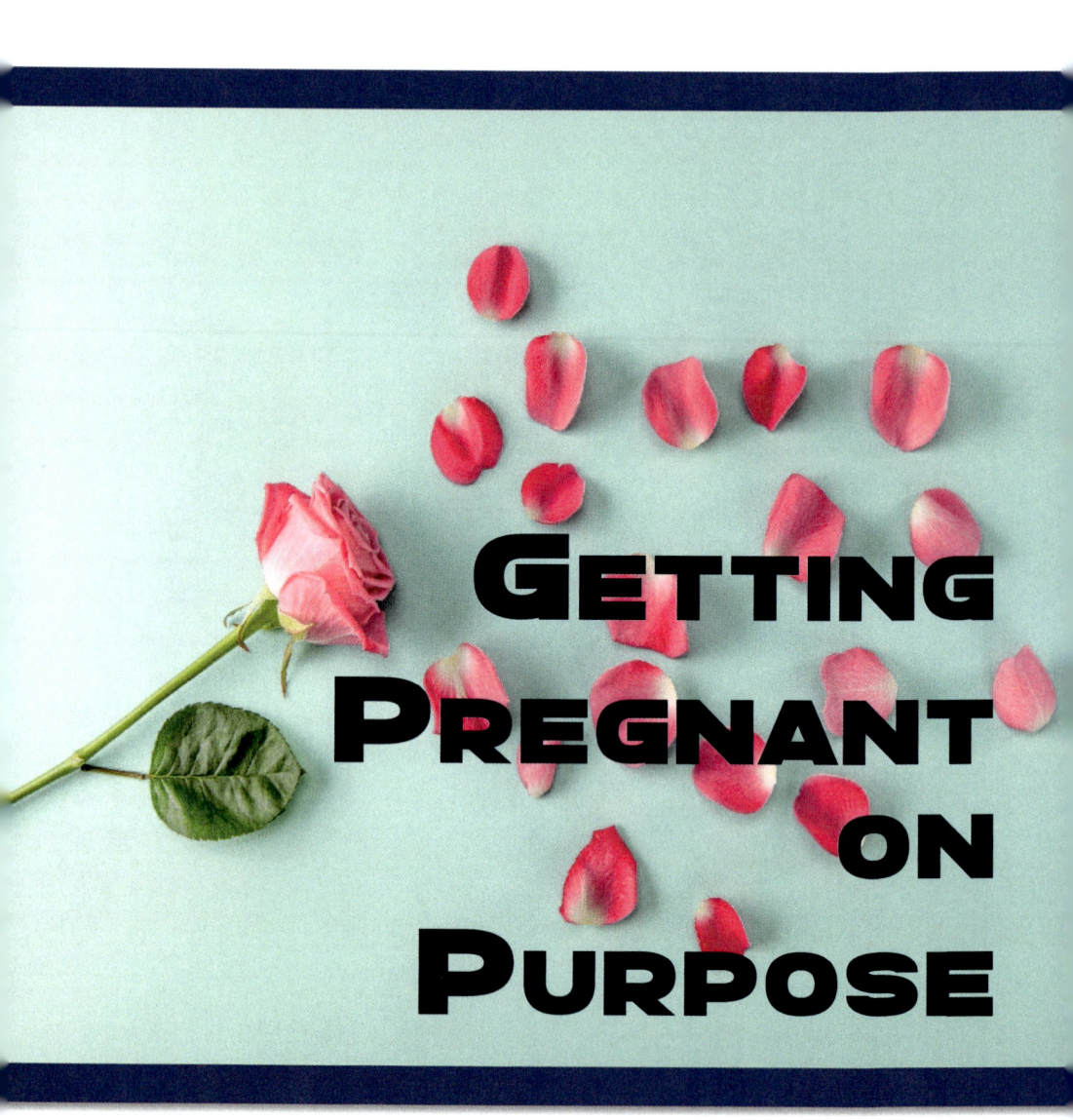

Getting Pregnant on Purpose

The Lord. The Lover. The Life Coach. SERIES™

ADVENTURE BEGINS

Getting pregnant on purpose – spiritually or physically is about desiring life, and life comes from God. But something has gone very wrong with this desire now. It has become warped and toxic for many. As human beings, we are born into sin from the DNA that was passed down to us from Adam and Eve, for God said, **"From dust you were taken, and to dust you shall return."** Dust refers to the word, 'earth' as in reddish clay mud, which comes from the word, 'adamah,' when God gave Adam his name.

In the beginning, the earth and everything in it was blessed by God who created it. Over time, the earth, the mud, the ground that yielded good fruit and provisions for humans became cursed by the decisions of humans. Adam and Eve first chose not to believe God, and instead they believed Satan and his satanic forces. They chose to act upon their beliefs and because of their choices, the ground was cursed. Remember, the ground was

Pregnant on Purpose

the earth from which man was created. Now, *"Houston, we have a problem."*

This is a big problem! Why is this such a big deal? Because God knows something we don't know. God's knowledge is greater than ours. His ways are not our ways; His thoughts are not our thoughts. The creature can never be greater than the Creator. The Word of God tells us in ***I John 3:4, "Whosoever committeth sin transgresseth also the law: for sin is the transgression of the law."***

The laws of the universe are now unable to operate properly because law has been broken. The perfect schematic of love and life and living in the presence of God's glory has now been tampered with. It is as if someone planted a virus in our computer's hard drive, and over time, the whole system, the files, directories, and programming are completely corrupt. The software, hardware, and the environment are all severely damaged goods. There is now intimate knowledge of both good and evil in the same being.

God our Father, the source of truth, being the Alpha and Omega, which is to say the creator of the beginning and the knower of the end of all

The Lord. The Lover. The Life Coach.
SERIES™

things, He knew that this was going to happen. But this, what you see today, was never His Plan. God had something greater in mind for you. His thoughts have always been and will always be higher than yours.

    Our Father God has always had a Plan that was higher than ours. His desire has always been that we are able to live in His presence, bask in His Glory, feed and care for ourselves and fellow man, and respect each other. God wanted us to enjoy ourselves in His creation while we held our dominion intact together as man and woman. His will is that we have the power to make choices and decide like Him. God knew that this was possible even from the beginning if we would choose to do so. His Purpose has always been about blessing humanity, not cursing it.

    This is still His Plan today. That's why Jesus Christ came to earth to set the story straight to us about God and His Providential Plan. All of this that we have seen in between the creation and now and even up until the end of time as we know it, came about because of what man decided to do, not because of what God wanted. God didn't choose this. Man did. But God has the Plan of

Pregnant on Purpose

The Lord. The Lover. The Life Coach.
SERIES™

deliverance because of His love. His deliverance plan was already set in motion before we got here. So you see, the story is much bigger than us. The story is about GOD WITH US. It is God revealing Himself to us. This is the Gospel of God!

Who Can Become Pregnant?

During a time of unprecedented challenge, trial, or change, like we are going through today, if a Believer wants to get pregnant on purpose, the man or woman who is whole and holy is the best candidate to carry out a pregnancy to full term. Desiring God's brilliant purpose for your life means becoming whole in the process. At every stage in life, no matter how old we get, Believers are to understand that we continually need and desire God as our Source of life, truth, completeness. It's God's provision for us!

We are continuously becoming whole and holy. We are not automatically born into the world whole. We have issues. Remember in the previous chapter we saw that when sin came, it transgressed the law – which means it broke the law of harmony that existed in the universe between God and man. The state that man is born into is a product of our human predecessors, Adam and Eve.

Psalm 51:5
Behold, I was shapen in iniquity; and in sin did my mother conceive me.

Ecclesiastes 7:20
For there is not a just man upon earth, that doeth good, and sinneth not.

Romans 3:10, 23
As it is written, There is none righteous, no, not one . . . For all have sinned, and come short of the glory of God;

Romans 5:8, 12
But God commendeth his love toward us, in that, while we were yet sinners, Christ died for us . . . Wherefore, as by one man sin entered into the world, and death by sin; and so death passed upon all men, for that all have sinned:

Psalm 14:1
The fool hath said in his heart, There is no God. They are corrupt, they have done abominable works, there is none that doeth good.

Romans 8:10
And if Christ be in you, the body is dead because of sin; but the Spirit is life because of righteousness.

The Lord. The Lover. The Life Coach.
SERIES™

1 John 1:8-10
If we say that we have no sin, we deceive ourselves, and the truth is not in us. If we confess our sins, he is faithful and just to forgive us our sins, and to cleanse us from all unrighteousness. If we say that we have not sinned, we make him a liar, and his word is not in us.

In sin, one does not grow to reach her full potential. The only way to grow is to become alive to Christ, the One who gives us the seed to grow – even to eternal life.

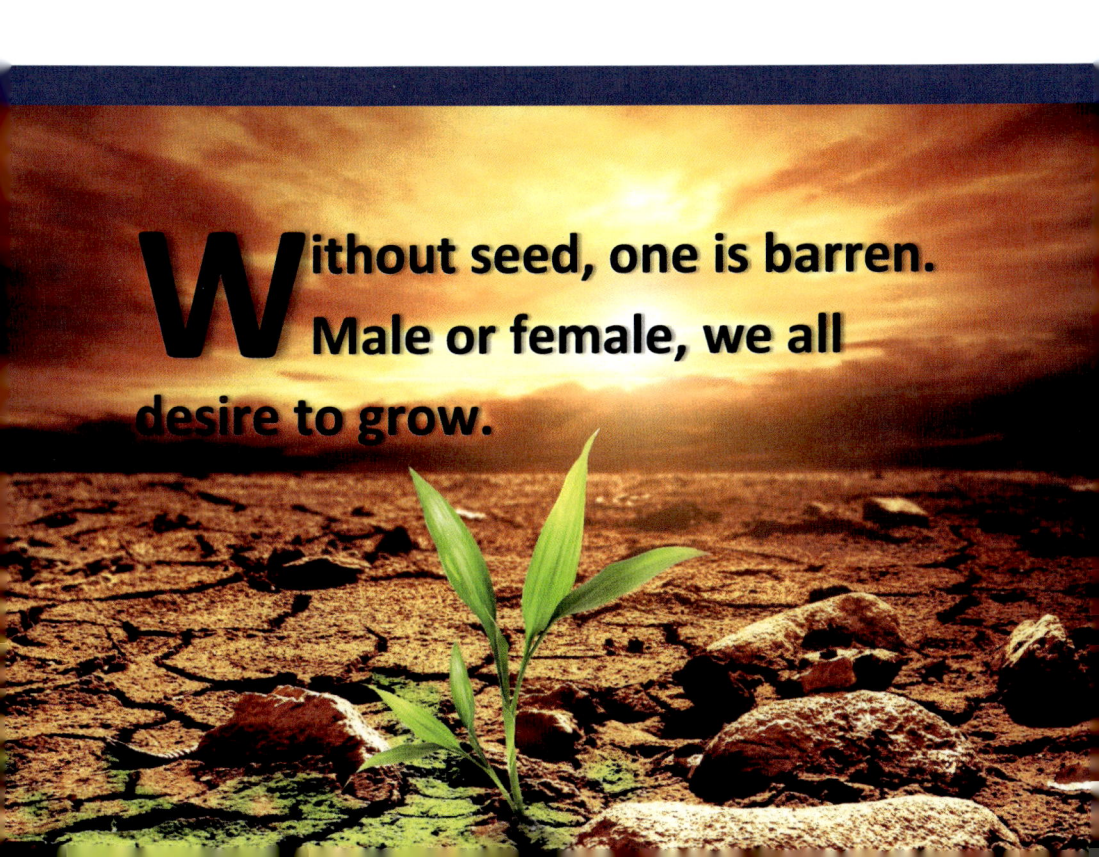

Without seed, one is barren. Male or female, we all desire to grow.

The image of God – that we were created with is that seed to grow! The capacity is in us before we are even born! The issue is not everyone wants to give birth to that seed. We are created in God's image. God is man's identity-carrier; we get our spiritual DNA from Him. But man at some point or another, chooses whether or not to accept this Spiritual Identity.

This is what it means to come into the knowledge of who you are in Christ. It is the most important decision you will ever have in life. Once you come into this revelation of who God is, and who you are in Him, your whole life is built upon this truth. It is the truth that you are created in God's image before you are even born. Before you stepped foot on planet earth, you were a seed in the heart of God. He desired YOU! Protect your seed. Stand guard over it by becoming WHOLE and HOLY! The man or woman who seeks God for wholeness and holiness is the one who is ready to become pregnant ON PURPOSE.

The Lord. The Lover. The Life Coach.
SERIES™

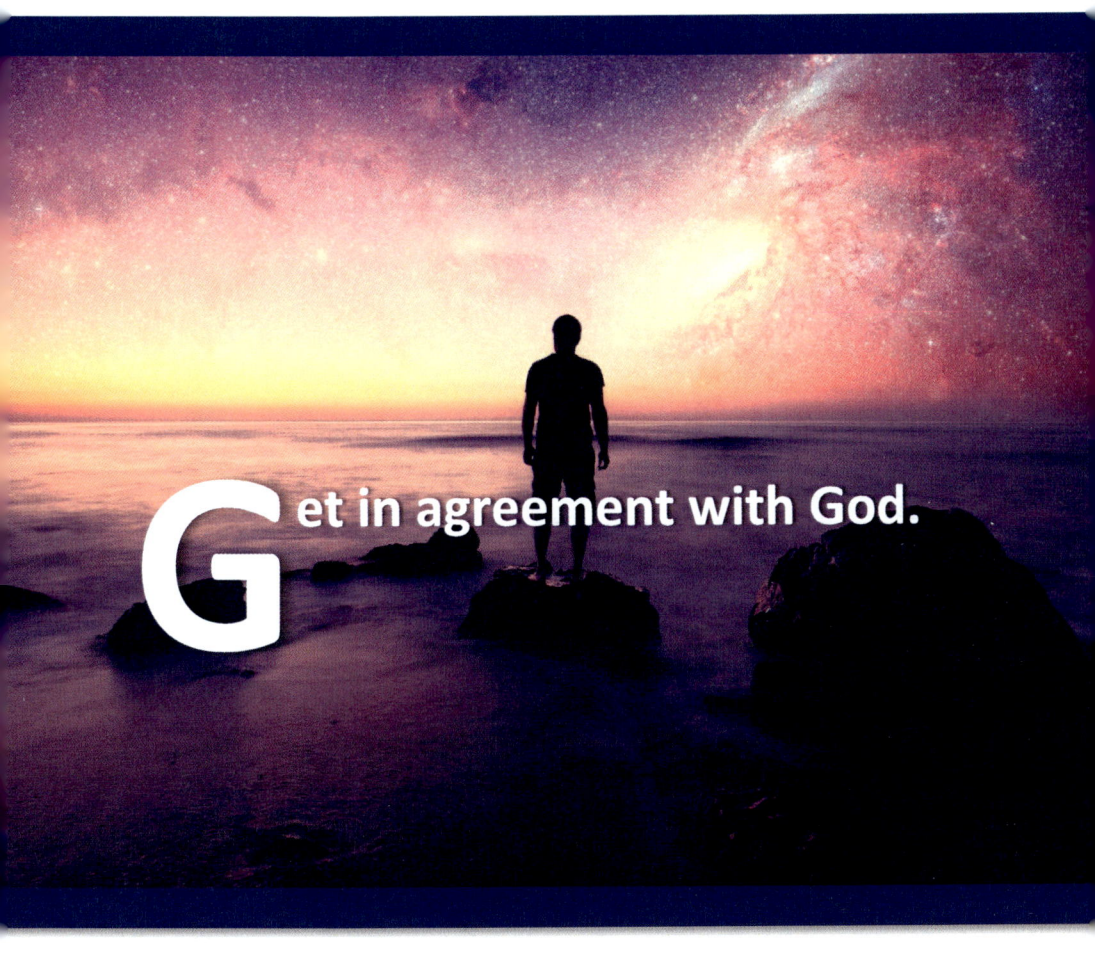

Get in agreement with God.

I n the next two chapters, I'll share practical wisdom, things you can do to check that your heart is pure towards God, yourself, and others. This opens you up to become pregnant on purpose – to conceive and carry God's brilliant plan for your life to full-term. Before closing, I'll give you 7 key concepts to seeing brilliance begin to manifest in your life using God's Word.

Pregnant on Purpose

Reflections

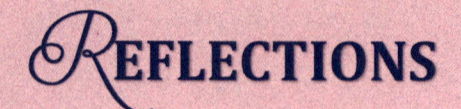

How is getting **pregnant on purpose** becoming an adventure?

Or is it?

How engaged are you in becoming pregnant?

How have you decided to use this exploration time and workbook?

Divorcing Religion and Dating Christ

Are You on Spiritual Birth Control?

One of the biggest hindrances to getting spiritually pregnant with God's brilliant purpose for your life is taking on things that hinder love and truth from taking root in your heart. Things like hypocrisy, false humility, and fake religious piety (what I call religiosity) are just a few of the things that work like birth control and contraceptives to hinder love and truth. These are why Jesus repeatedly rebuked the Jews.

Religiosity is what is shown when you do things for God out of obligation and a sense of work. When you say with your mouth that you desire God, love God, and honor Him, but with your heart, you are far from Him and you really don't want to become closer to Him, that's hypocritical. It is what happens when one's motives are not pure. Sometimes, you can tell when a person's motives are not pure. For example, when we refuse to love others, regardless of their background and where they come from, this is a conditional love not a pure love. You refuse to show mercy and compassion. You walk in selfish pride and don't want to be corrected by anyone. You really don't want to hear the truth about yourself from others who have to live or work with you. These are just examples of things that work like contraceptives against the motives of genuine love and truth.

Genuine love and truth are the behaviors that Jesus showed us. At the same time that Jesus showed us love, He also showed us disruption where man's behavior came against the truth of who God really is. When it came to representing God's love and God's truth at the same time, Jesus was there to give the proper example of God's identity. He even turned the tables and shut the mouths of the religious fakers and shakers of that day. Jesus gave us indicators and hints of what it means to walk in God's truth and love at the same time. This was His purpose for coming – to testify to the truth about who God really is ***(John 18:37)***.

This is not a book about end times, but I think it is no coincidence that we are seeing a number of things on earth now that reflect the last days described in the book of Revelations. These things are giving witness to the truth about God's Word; they are showing us what God knew way before we got here so that we might believe God and agree with what Jesus has taught us.

God addresses what happens to the impious, easily influenced by outward displays of affection for God, but one who is internally stiff-necked, indifferent, or self-righteous. This is a person who has eyes, but does not want to see – the truth about what God is revealing. **They have other motivations for following God,** for example, stealing the hearts of the people for their own advancement. This is what idolatry does; it removes the focus off God and onto personal motives. People who practice such motives tend to closely associate religion with fake humility, not pure humility. Now is the time to look inside our hearts, especially if we love God. This book is a exploration tool to assist you.

2020 has been a heck of an adventure to say the least. For Believers in Christ and those who are not, this year has felt like one hell of a rollercoaster ride. As the new year approaches, let's consider leaving some things behind us, like cutting the cords of religion and the idols of our culture. Instead, let's fall earnestly in love with God again.

The Lord. The Lover. The Life Coach. SERIES™

If you're going to mass, church, or synagogue just because it's the right thing to do, you might as well stay home. There's no love in that. If you're on the prayer line because it's prayer time, but you stir up negativity or mess, you might as well hang up the phone. There's no truth in that. If you're giving to the poor because it's good PR and gets your business or brand noticed, then don't expect anything else from God; you're already getting a tax deduction. There's no love in that. And if you're preaching, teaching, and serving others in ministry because it strokes your ego, raises your self-esteem, and boosts your confidence levels, then you might as well visit a bar, drink a bottle of Jack Daniel's, and dance naked on the tables. Sit down somewhere. There's no truth or love in that.

The Lord. The Lover. The Life Coach.
SERIES™

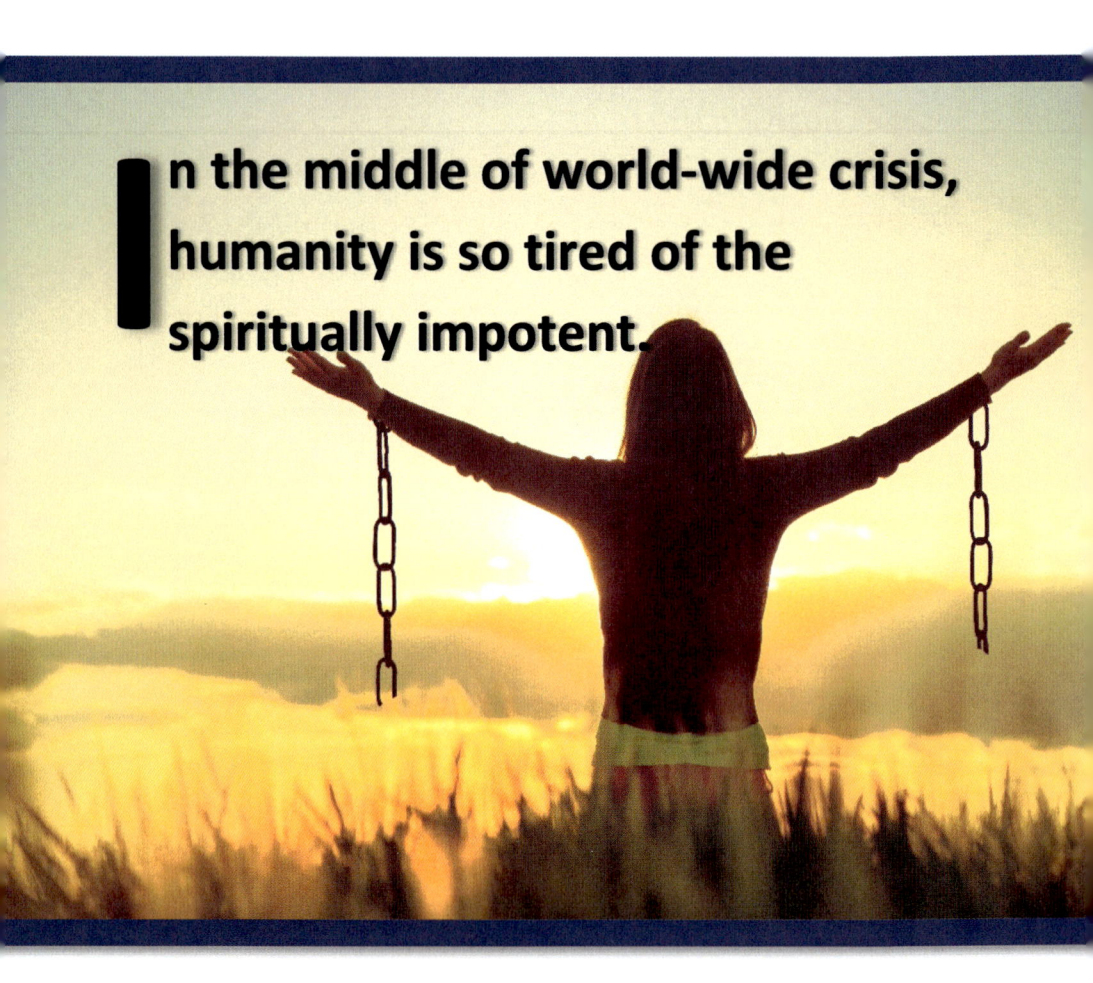

> In the middle of world-wide crisis, humanity is so tired of the spiritually impotent.

Spiritual Impotence

If you wear Christianity like it's a badge at a paid conference with a lanyard around your neck, then you might as well had kept your money and stayed at home. God is actively alive and well in the Body of Believers today, and He takes delight in

Pregnant on Purpose

The Lord. The Lover. The Life Coach. SERIES™

living inside of us. if you do not trust Him enough to humble yourself before Him, and let Him use you in body, soul, and spirit, then you might as well sit down somewhere. Christ Jesus does you no good.

Listen up people, Holiness is not an act.

It's an *aspiration.*

Listen up world, Christ is not the problem.

He's the *solution.*

Listen up unsaved, God is not boring;

He's the Life of the party. In fact, ***He's the One who invited you.***

Pregnant on Purpose

The Lord. The Lover. The Life Coach.
SERIES™

Listen up, everybody,

Christianity is not a ritual. It's a *real relationship - like the one you want to have with the love of your life!*

Some of us have a relationship status with God like the one we see posted on Facebook, Instagram, and Twitter.

Ours says:

♥ *It's complicated.*

But is being Christian really that complicated? Or, have we just made it seem that way because we do things like: we don't know who we are? We put crazy people on pedestals? We encourage drama? We do anything for a dollar? We refuse to take responsibility for those who cannot care for themselves?

Loving God and being a replica of Him to change the world is really not that complicated

Pregnant on Purpose

according to Jesus. He says, *"Take my yoke upon you and learn of me, for my yoke is easy and my burden is light."*

When are you going to fall in love with God like a Lover? What will it take you to be drawn into Him like He's drawn into you?

He dances over you at night, and gives you Light in darkness. He feeds your hunger for love and fulfills your thirsty soul. He waters your ground when your land is dry; and every time evil has sought to touch you, steal from you, or destroy you and take what is yours, the Lord has made a covenant with you, His people. We have access to dispatch thousands upon thousands of angels who are given a mandate to kick a** and take names in this life and the one to come.

If we do not know how to exercise our God-given right to have dominion in our own home, city, country, nation, or in our own space, then that is not the failure of God; perhaps we need to re-examine our relationships - not just our relationship with God, but our relationship with the things that drive us. What have we given our hearts to? Who are we dating with our desires?

And who are we in bed with to make us joyful and content?

As Believers, we do not deny that trials and strife exist; the struggle is real. But our God is more real. His truth triumphs. His love speaks volumes as He makes His Word come alive through Christ.

He's not just God when we're on the mountaintop flexing our muscles in dominion. He's also God in the valley of our down-and-out speaking life to dry bones.

In these trying times, who are we needing to leave behind? What are we needing to cut loose? What is that inside of us which is keeping us from excelling and experiencing God's very best for our lives? How could this same power or principality be hindering us from moving forward with others?

I want to leave behind the impious me. I want to cut the umbilical cord of any remaining traces of un-pure religion. I want to push forward and present a me that genuinely desires to show forth the love and power of Christ to God, myself, and others.

Let's do it together. Won't you join me?

Divorcing religion and dating Christ!

The Lord. The Lover. The Life Coach.
SERIES™

Galatians 5:22-26
22 But the fruit of the Spirit is love, joy, peace, longsuffering, gentleness, goodness, faith,
23 Meekness, temperance: against such there is no law.
24 And they that are Christ's have crucified the flesh with the affections and lusts.
25 If we live in the Spirit, let us also walk in the Spirit.
26 Let us not be desirous of vain glory, provoking one another, envying one another.

If you really want to see change in your spiritual life, then get off the spiritual birth control. Begin applying the wisdom of God in every area, even as a single woman. Wisdom will carry you into your future. Read on – there's more single girl power – real practical wisdom that can and will elevate you when applied to your day-to-day life.

Applying Wisdom

What are you willing to do in order to remove hindrances to your God-given purpose and brilliance?

What needs to change?
About yourself?
About religion?
About others?

Don't Sleep with my Husband

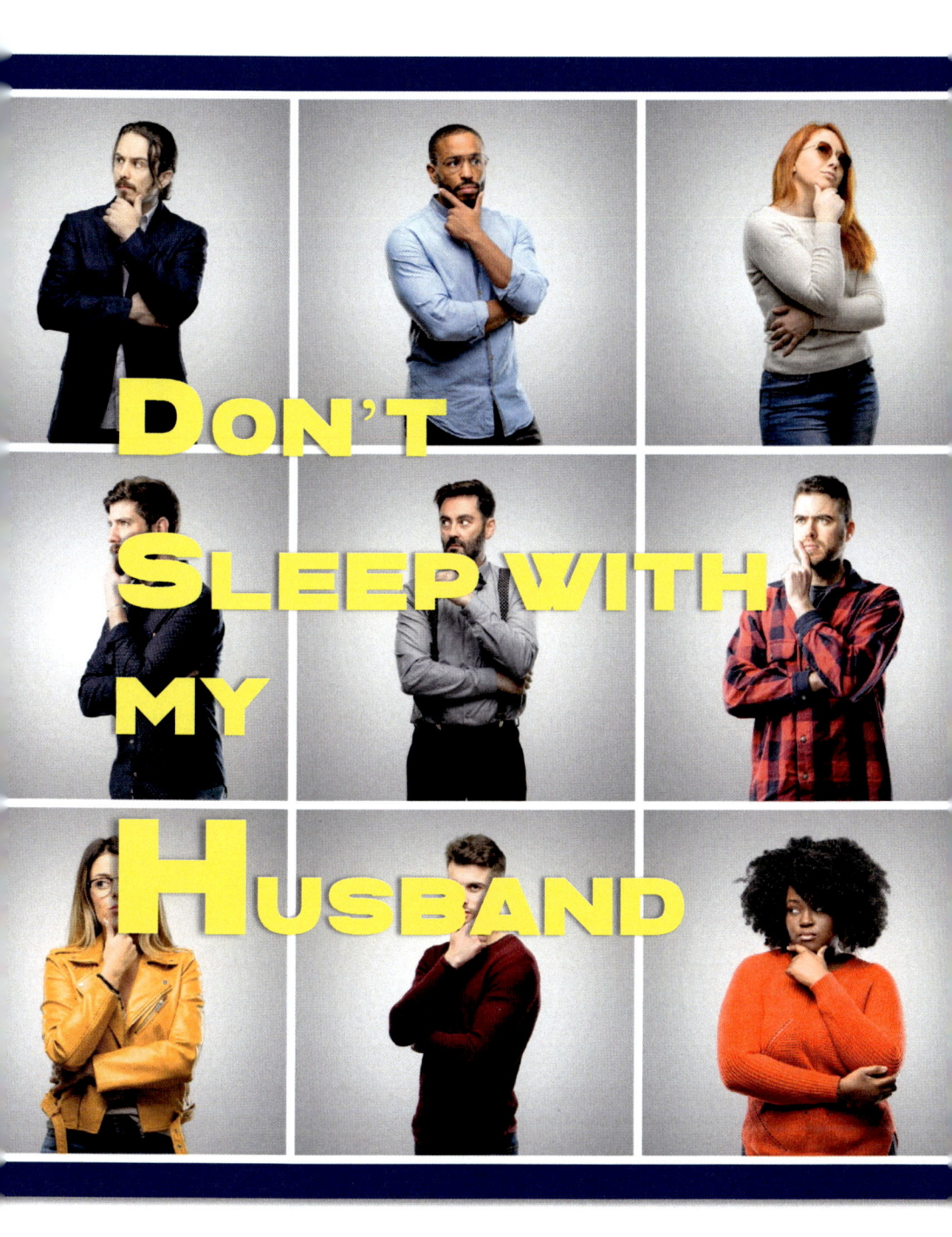

Pregnant on Purpose

The Lord. The Lover. The Life Coach.
SERIES™

DON'T SLEEP WITH MY HUSBAND

My Purpose Partner

Women have been sleeping with each other's husbands for centuries, creating hell-pots of confusion and distress. Since before the days of Rachel and Leah (the daughters of Laban and brides to Jacob in the Bible) women have been breaking each other's hearts. I saw it with my grandmother, my mother, and many others around me share the same issue. We mourned over our men, whether they deserved our love or not. This is because we want to see them as more than just sex partners; we desire Purpose Partners.

Come on, Ladies, when it comes to our husbands, we should all consider ourselves sisters. It doesn't matter where we come from, or what side of the fence we live on, the business and

The Lord. The Lover. The Life Coach.
SERIES™

calling of being a woman demands that we respect certain sacred laws. Sacred laws are those that I believe were designed for life and harmony. As females from the same species, we should love each other and see each other as sisters. Not only that, we should see our spouses as Purpose Partners.

We talk about the challenges we have with the men in our lives; we talk about our disappointments with the way they act, think, and behave. But the truth is this: God made us to fit! We are counterparts of one another – a common species – to fit men, physically, spiritually, emotionally, and mentally. God didn't make us mistakes to one another. He made us counterparts to POP into place just like pieces of a puzzle that fit together!

Some puzzles are more complex than others and take more time to figure out how the pieces come together, but sooner or later – if they came out of the right box, the pieces do fit. Partners of Purpose are those spouses that are not only in your life for the obvious external rewards, but they are also there to help shape the gifts inside of you that others may not be able to see. They help bring out

Pregnant on Purpose

your God-given brilliance. Men who desire to marry should also want to marry a woman who is a Partner of Purpose. A woman who is a Partner of Purpose will not only nurture the physical, but she is capable of nurturing a mans needs for purpose.

Taking the Oath of Sisterhood

A wise person once said, "Don't complain about a problem that you're unwilling to solve." So today, is my day to solve this problem, in my own way, in my own time, and in my own space.

Honoring this pledge of Sisterhood is my solution to the problem of heartbreak amongst sisters. It's a heart-to-heart woman-to-woman covered in the blood covenant promise that I will never sleep with your husband!

I'm asking women everywhere, no, shall I dare say, I am decreeing everywhere, that you will never sleep with mine!

True sisterhood is the cure for infidelity. It will stop any man from being unfaithful and destroying his family. It will save children's lives and reduce the premature death rate. It will decrease teenage pregnancy and reduce the risk of life-threatening illnesses. I am convinced that sisterhood will save, protect, and prosper mankind. It will preserve the dignity of our younger men, and resurrect all that's good and once thought dead in the hearts of our older men.

I watched my grandfather grieve himself to death while living with his mistress. I watched an anointed pastor with a beautiful family, thriving congregation lose everything of value after committing adultery. Sisters, we can fix this when we all band together. Taking the pledge of Sisterhood is not the panacea for saving failed marriages because we know that sometimes divorce is necessary. But living by the principles of Sisterhood is the answer to preventing the heartbreak of infidelity, something that is 100% preventable - for the most part - if women would love and respect each other as sisters.

It's so amazing how something so simple can have such an amazing impact. I believe with God, all things are possible, even an amazing spouse and great monogamous lovemaking is possible with God! That's what I'm believing God for! How about you? Why not believe God for an amazing resurrected life with the men on the planet? What about changing the culture when it comes to the men in our lives? What about improving the marriage bed – honoring it and un-defiling it? If sisters would work together on issues like this, all things are possible to them that believe! The problem is many of us don't know how to live like we believe, can't connect with God, and don't know how to connect with our spouses. I found a wonderful Sisterhood Pledge online. Find one that you can believe in and practice, or better yet – write your own below.

      Just a note of caution: as I have done in my other teachings, I have concentrated mostly on women. This is not because I believe that men are not in need of assistance; it's quite the contrary. However, my assignment in this workbook is to coach women toward their destiny using the application of God's Word. I believe an intimate relationship with God is highly effectual in transforming the dreams and visions of women into reality when we apply ourselves to an intimate walk with Him as a way of life. Know, however, that all of the principles herein can also easily apply to men and sons who are maturing in the faith.

Pregnant on Purpose

Oath of Sisterhood

_____
_____
_____
_____
_____
_____
_____
_____
_____
_____
_____
_____
_____
_____
_____

Share a Sisterhood Pledge that you believe in, or create your own here.

What are your strongest internal thoughts about women and sisterhood? What are your thoughts about our purpose and men?

The Lord. The Lover. The Life Coach.
SERIES™

Take 1 day to focus on one concept covered in the next section. These are self-exploration tips that have guided my life on a daily basis. I try to spread them across a one week period to help build and reinforce good habits every day. These tips are taken from going deeper into Scripture during some of my most challenging times in life. I pray that you allow the Holy Spirit to teach you, coach you, and lead you into what HE wants you to know about getting Pregnant on Purpose in order to live out your full potential. May the Lord keep you, cause His face to shine upon you, and cause you to become full, overflowing in the things both natural and spiritual that He has just for you!

DAY 1

Knowing what you

Believe

The Lord. The Lover. The Life **Coach.**
SERIES™

DAY 1 – KNOW WHAT YOU BELIEVE

> Make a bold statement within yourself, and began to live it. Fall in love with God's truth and His love. Together, you'll make beautiful babies!

On January 12, I wrote out my **Pregnant on Purpose** faith confession before this book was written. This confession came as I spent the night with the Holy One and woke up having received His seed the next morning. On that next morning, I wrote:

I am fully accepted, beloved, cared for, and developed in WHO I am called to be and WHAT I am called to accomplish in this life and beyond because of my Father, God, His Christ and Holy Spirit. This means that I am fully accepted, beloved, cared for, and developed in WHO I am, WHOSE I am, and WHAT is my destiny in this life and beyond. I am in love, enthused, engaged, and empowered on purpose because my foundation is: Jesus, who is God's expressed character, nature, and Word. His

The Lord. The Lover. The Life Coach.
SERIES™

Holy Spirit who is God's expressed will, wisdom, and work, and God Himself, who is my Creator, my identity bearer, and my Father, my Source of Truth has taken the time to draw me near to Him that I might personally come to know Him as Lover and Revealer. He revealed Himself to me as Light in the darkness so that I would know who I am and in doing so, know Him as my "I Am."

Therefore, my desire is to love the Lord my God, with all my heart, with all my soul (which is my mind, will, emotions, intellect, inspiration, imagination, desires, drive, development, and libido). With all my strength, I desire to become transformed into God's image that I might love others more, and more healthily love myself. As I am intimate with God, I come to know Him as Love and Truth, then I can demonstrate and deliver the same to others.

My life and Somebody else's is about to change for the better!

℘REGNANT ON PURPOSE CONFESSION

_____
_____
_____
_____
_____
_____
_____
_____
_____
_____
_____
_____
_____

What's your confession concerning birthing out God's brilliant plan for you?

How can you live out your bold statement of faith through love and truth at the same time? What does this mean for you?

DAY 2
Checking your heart

The Lord. The Lover. The Life Coach.
SERIES™

DAY 2 – CHECK YOUR HEART

> **To help realize God's brilliant plan for your life, prepare to be drawn spiritually. Consider taking about 30-minutes to self-explore one of these tips each day.**

1. SET your faith.

Believers WIN not because they are perfect, but because they desire to embrace the truth about who God really is. If you have stumbled across this book, know that Jesus, the King of Glory has come to live in your house this season. Welcome HIM in. He wants to show you the truth about who God really is. Turn your face like a flint towards heaven. **(Isaiah 50:7)**

2. COME ready to fall in love with God.

Open your arms in complete surrender to GOD as your first LOVE. This book was written to women, but men desire to fall in love too. Man, as the first created being on earth, has deep need to love and be loved. I believe that a man can love properly if he is in a real relationship with God, where he believes and trusts God, and loves others. I believe this because God made man in His image, and God is love. *(1 John 4:7-21)*

3. THROW OUT presumptions.

Don't assume God's going to move a certain way. Just consult HIM for what is on your mind and what is in your heart, like you would consult someone with whom you are in love. *(Numbers 15:30)*

4. TRUST the work of Christ.

He brings you to GOD and serves as your only GOD. Worship, honor, and adore HIM only. Very important not to insult GOD by placing your faith in things or people. People make mistakes. This is why it's necessary to trust the work of Christ in order to forgive mistakes, both your own and those of others. Not only do you trust GOD, but also trust His process. GOD has instituted the law because

Pregnant on Purpose

He knew it was necessary, so respect law and order because it honors GOD. Where law and order become immoral, GOD help us! The way of both truth and love is the way of Christ. He knows the way in which GOD wants to take you. *(Philippians 3: 4-7)*

5. QUIET your soul.

Increase your peace level. Remove any wounds that are hindering you from experiencing peace. Sanctify your imagination to inspire your soul. Ask yourself what is it that you like to do that brings you to GOD's face? Think on those things, and do them! Contend, if you must, for your peace level. *(Isaiah 26:3)*

6. LOVE, LOVE, LOVE.

A focus on Purpose demands a look at love and motivations. In this book, when I refer to a Purpose Partner for the Single Person, I am speaking of relationships with significant others or friends who become significant others. This calls for a review on what you

Pregnant on Purpose

really know about love. I found a wonderful chart on FTD.com, the floral company, that speaks of the types of love that I'm focusing on in this book on purpose. Go to this website and take a look at the chart they have posted on the types of love: https://www.ftd.com/blog/give/types-of-love. From the chart, you can see that there are primarily three focuses upon which one might look at another person who is considered a significant other in one's life. These 3 types of love are: ludus (playful love), eros (romantic love) and pragma (enduring love) and I believe that all of these types work together specifically when one is in a relationship with a significant other who is a Purpose Partner. Not all people we call significant others are Purpose Partners for us. It's important to me that a significant other Purpose Partner relationship where I am living in love with a person will exhibit all three of these types of love. If all three of these do not exist in a significant other relationship, then that relationship might be a friendship or a family relationship, but not a significant other relationship. Why am I focusing on significant other relationships? Because it is my belief that if a significant other relationship does not entail a Purpose Partner, then it is a waste of time, because the birthing that takes place from the relationship is not of purpose.

Now, does that mean that we only have purpose with significant others? No, there are family relationships with which we have purpose. There are also friendships with which we have purpose. Those are special relationships too! But in this book, I'm speaking of becoming pregnant on purpose by becoming intimate with God and my focus is to show you the parallel by showing you what it looks like when you are in a relationship with the Love of your life. So to understand how to properly love the love of your life, you need to understand ludus (playful love), eros (romantic love), and pragma (enduring love) if the relationship is going to be leading to becoming pregnant, fruitful, or productive. Therefore, it follows that you should know and understand all three of those types of love.

The other types of love not spoken about in this book are a given for relationships with any individuals not just significant others. Check out the link just shared on FTD.com to make sure that you are building healthy loving relationships with all individuals if you plan to become spiritually pregnant by God. You will need to have a heart for those kinds of love as well. Seek to love others in the same manner as you would love and care for yourself and loved ones. We all have difficulty loving others unconditionally. Seek to understand what you have within you from God so that you can give more of yourself like God gives you. Learn to love another person genuinely without cynicism and judgment, even when they don't deserve it. When people do wrong, judge their behavior, and not their heart. This means, take the appropriate action, and still love the person. *(Isaiah 26:3)*

7. PAY ATTENTION to your life.

Your dreams, visions, and aspirations tell you something. Run them through God's Word, and especially His character. This means searching Him out. How do you search God out? Get in His Presence in His Word, pray, and listen to your innermost convictions about truth and love working together.

Pay attention when something repeatedly comes up: a word, a phrase, a picture, or a thought whether you think it is a good dream or not. A dream or vision for your life will make you more selective about what you allow yourself to watch, hear, taste, smell, or touch. In other words, a vision or dream from your potential will sharpen your five spiritual senses. You will want to test your dreams and visions, examining them more fully for what is real for you and what is not. My actions also tell me a lot about where my heart is on a particular matter. If I am angry, if I lash out, if I am not being honest with myself, sometimes these things visit me in my dreams. Write things down and lay them at God's feet in prayer, trusting the character of Christ to teach you things that you need to know about life and godliness. Sometimes we seek the thoughts of others whom we have come to know and trust, and that's okay; the Bible says there is wisdom in a multitude of counsel and coaching may also be a great way to open up your space and gain clarity. *(Proverbs 11:14)*

Self-Check Assessment

Which one of these areas is most difficult for you? What limiting beliefs do you have that may be holding you back?

What's possible that you are beliving about God, about you, or about others that is causing you difficulty?

DAY 3

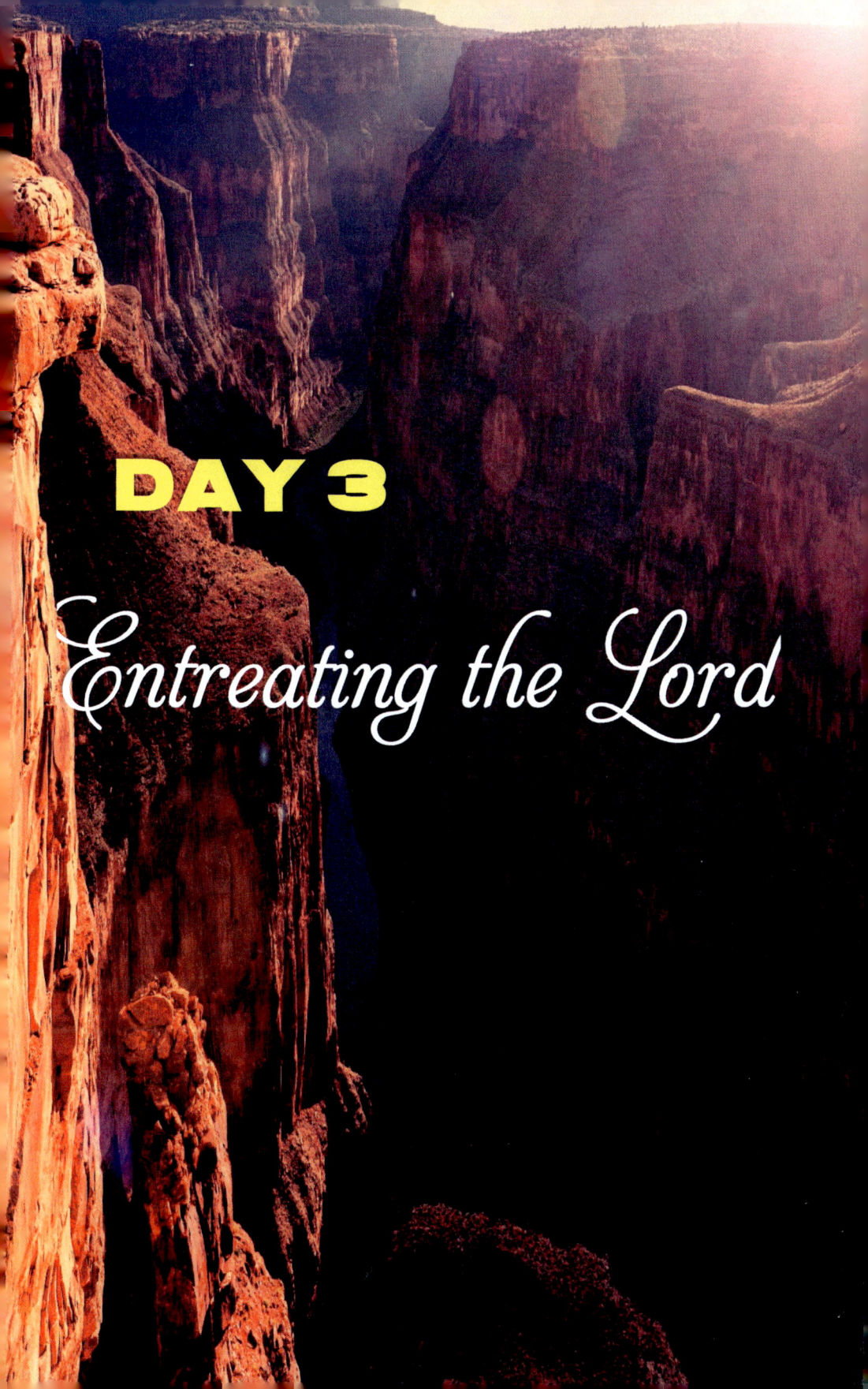

Entreating the Lord

DAY 3 – ENTREAT THE LORD

> **The wrong companion will keep you barren. But the right one will "entreat the Lord." When "PREGNANT ON PURPOSE," you need the kind of love that outlasts the night!**

If you are feeling barrenness or difficulty in conceiving, the secret to birthing is not in you, but in God! Your assignment is to lie down with God, and open up to receive His secrets. Three things to embrace as you lie down with God:

1. You've got to be willing to let Him love on you.
2. You got to be willing to love others no matter what you think about them; love them like He loves you.
3. You've got to be willing to seek His Wisdom like you're looking for the Love of your life.

The best way to become ready for Purpose is to become intimate with God first. Saturate yourself in His truth and His love. Practice these virtues on a daily basis

The Lord. The Lover. The Life Coach.
SERIES™

with the people around you, on your job, or in your community. See where you are in need of more maturity. See how fast you embrace producing fruit of the Spirit: love, joy, peace, faith, gentleness, meekness, kindness, longsuffering, and self-control, for example. This will help you see where you really are in the faith, and whether you are ready for a Purpose Partner. You don't have to be perfect to be a Purpose Partner; you just have to be willing.

Blessings for a powerful purposeful personal encounter with your true self first before God, and then when the time is right, a Partner of Purpose!

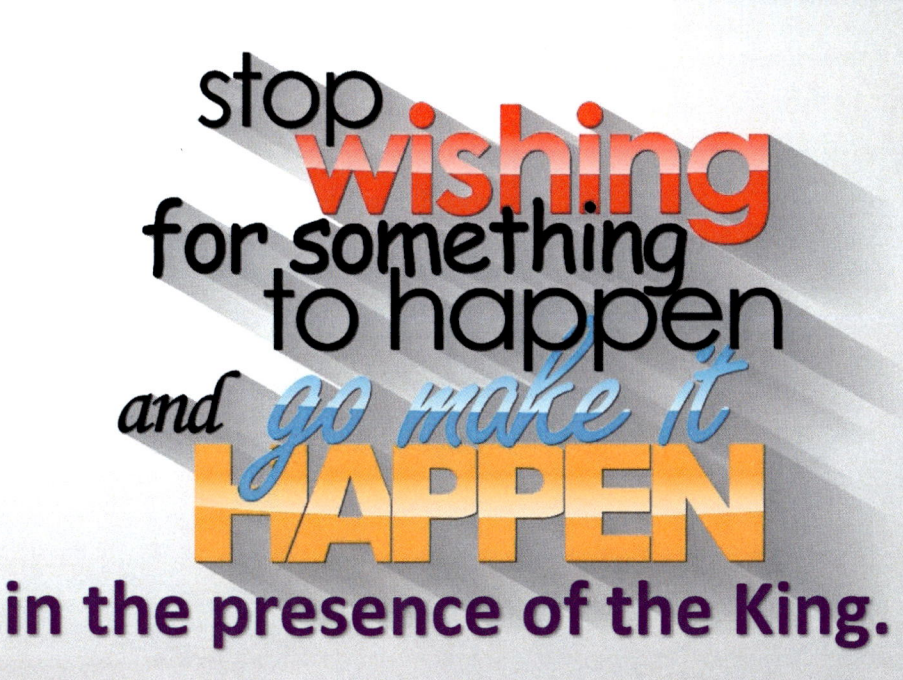

stop wishing for something to happen and go make it HAPPEN in the presence of the King.

Purpose Partner Entreaty

Examine your motivations on Purpose with another and ask:

"What are the ways in which I have experienced both love and truth with my Purpose Partner?
"What sacrifices are made with my Purpose Partner?"
"Which types of love do I identify with most in my Purpose Partner?

DAY 4

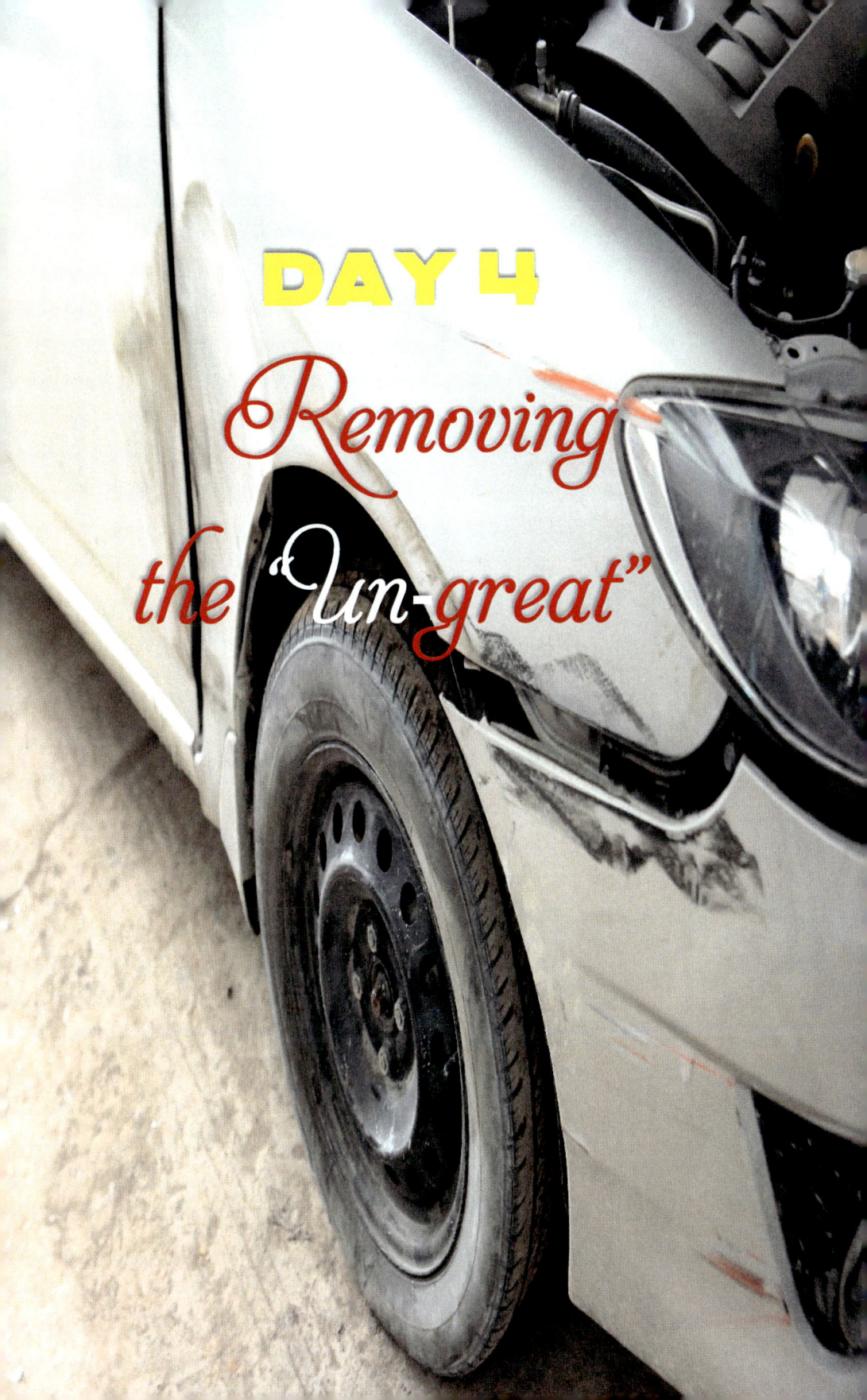

Removing the "Un-great"

The Lord. The Lover. The Life Coach.
SERIES™

DAY 4 – REMOVE THE 'UNGREAT'

> **I wasn't ready to meet a great Purpose Partner until I was ready to let go of the ungreat.**

I heard Steve Harvey say that his mom gave him the greatest advice. He said as a young man while he was still living at home with his mom, he kept resounding on an on about getting this new dream vehicle he had in mind. He saved for it, worked for it, and kept going on and on about how he was going to get it one day. His mom finally got tired of hearing him talk about it and said to him that he couldn't get a new one until he moved his old beat-up broken down junk car out of the middle of her driveway. This resonated with me. I didn't make myself available to meet a great Purpose Partner until I was ready to let go of those who were not interested in Purpose or ready for purpose.

This year, I met a great man online and we decided to try dating. This was the first real relationship that I had held since my divorce over

The Lord. The Lover. The Life Coach.
SERIES™

ten years ago. I tried dating very briefly in the past, but nothing ever worked out. This time is different. We are not looking to be engaged or married to each other, but God is still in our midst. We became true friends. We both love God and also love and respect each other. This is because we are both whole.

When you know and love yourself first, then you can know and love another. It is not possible to know and love another person until you know and love yourself in a healthy manner. That is the way dating should be.

John 4:14
But whosoever drinketh of the water that I shall give him shall never thirst; but the water that I shall give him shall be in him a well of water springing up into everlasting life.

Pregnant on Purpose

SEEKING INTIMACY

Who are you being seen by for intimacy? Why?

What are the deeper connections that you seek? How are you being honest to yourself and God about the desires and motivations you have for intimacy and purpose?

DAY 5

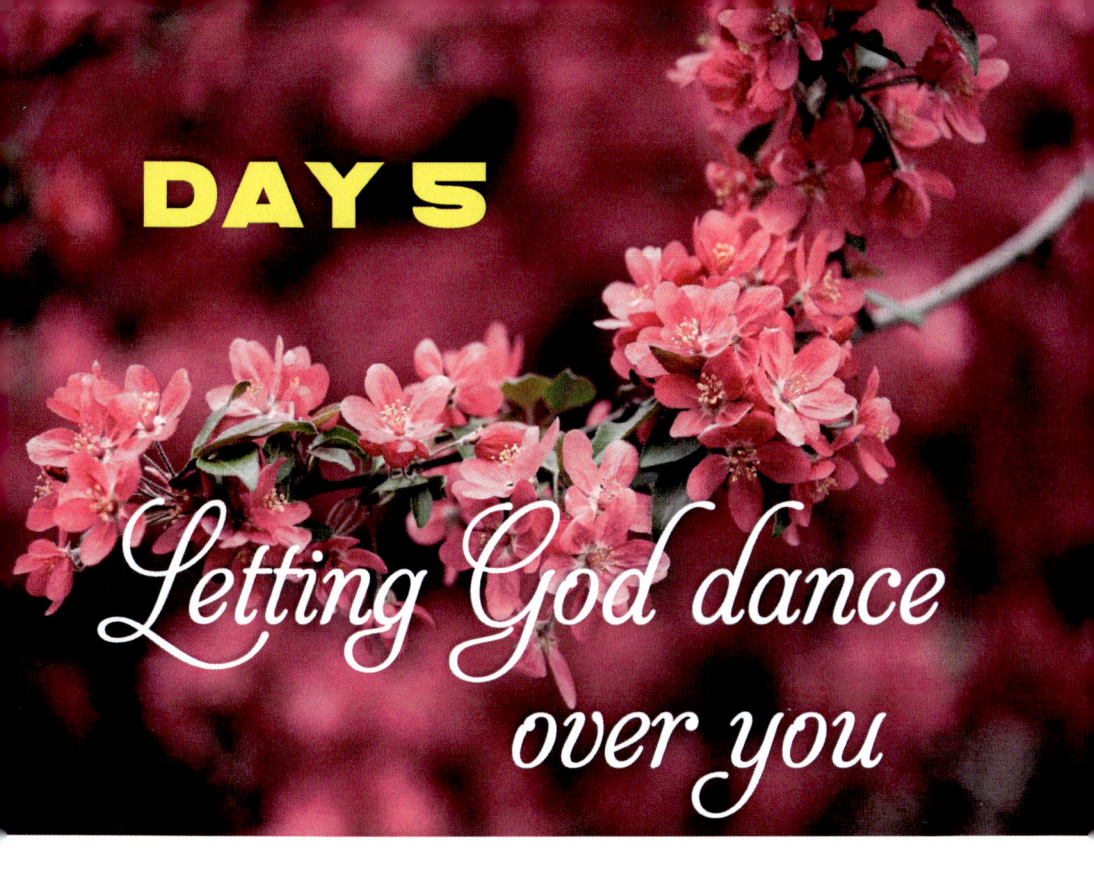

Letting God dance over you

DAY 5 – HE DANCES OVER YOU

Healing My Libido

Zephaniah 3:17
The Lord thy God in the midst of thee is mighty; he will save, he will rejoice over thee with joy; he will rest in his love, he will joy over thee with singing.

PREGNANT on PURPOSE

The Lord. The Lover. The Life Coach. SERIES™

In my loneliest times, God has reassured me that he would be a husband over me. He has ministered to me in all of my areas of need, including healing my libido. When you have been married, as I have, and then single again after marriage, adjusting to changes in your sexual life can a challenge.

Temptations can be tough, even painful and dangerous. It is important to realize that God knows and understands. His perspective is healing your soul entirely in wholeness and holiness. If you pull on your relationship with God as husband, He will romance you, dance over you, and bring you through faithfully. There is a yielding necessary on your part, but it's another opportunity to open yourself to the Lord. God responds to your opening up yourself to His Spirit.

He allows me to be healed in those areas and to continue to walk in wholeness and holiness. We don't have to go from pillar to post when we allow the Lord to dance over us.

Learning to Dance with God

How do you come boldly before God in time of need for everything, and not just for some things, even intimacy?

Where do you desire both wholeness and holiness in intimacy with God and with another?

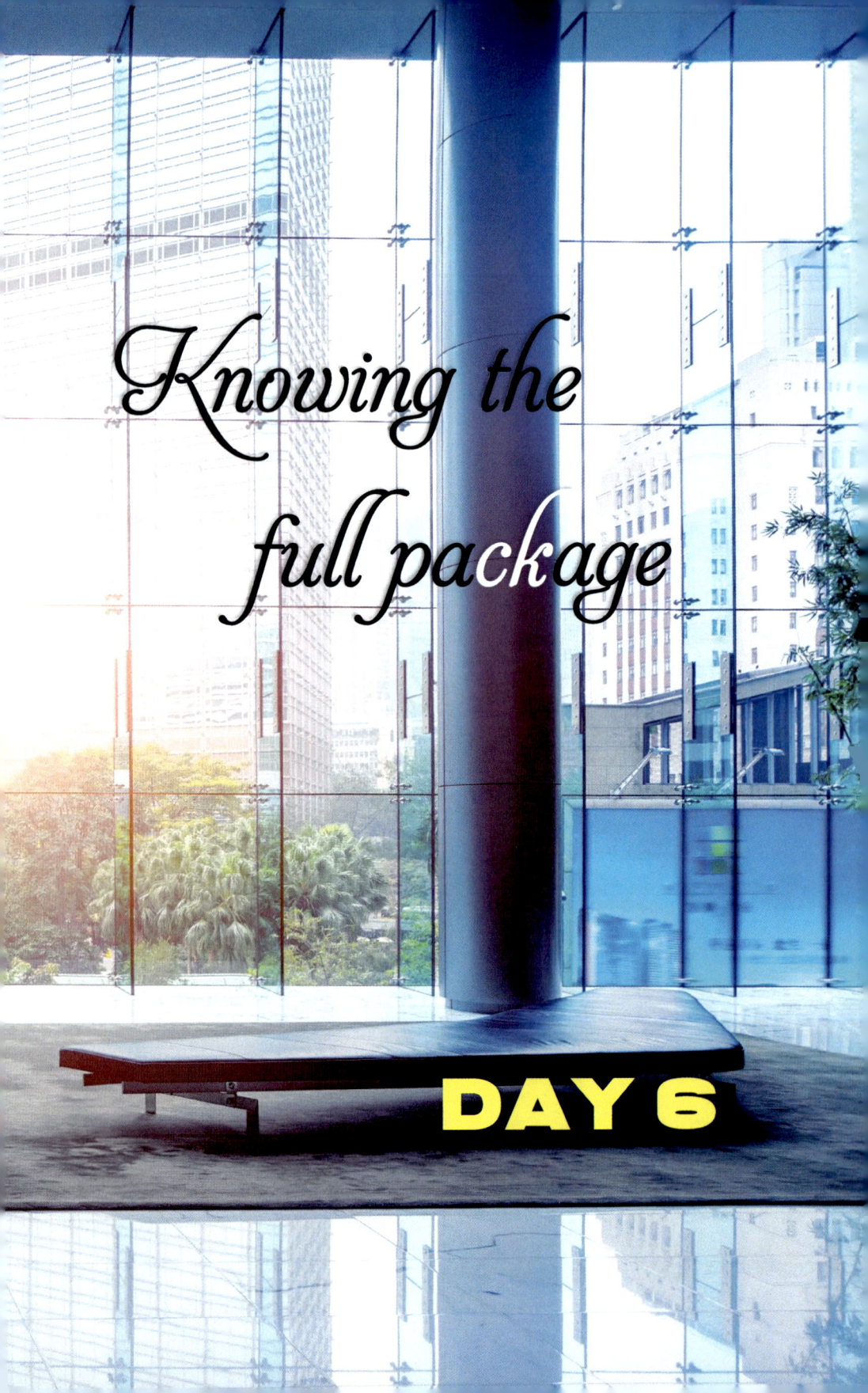

Knowing the full package

DAY 6

The Lord. The Lover. The Life Coach. SERIES™

DAY 6 – KNOWING THE FULL PACKAGE

Intimacy, Beauty, and Adventure

So many singles are turning people away because they are looking for "the full package." But would you know the full package if it was standing right in front of you?

> **We need to know the full package before we can receive the full package.**

- It's not looks!
- It's not sex!
- It's Intimacy, Beauty, & Adventure

For many years, I struggled to put into words just want it was that I was looking for in a relationship. Even after being saved, filled with the Spirit, I still couldn't express what it was that my soul was after in a relationship with a person. Then, it occurred to me if I didn't know or couldn't express my desires and needs clearly, then how could I expect another person? Entering into the secret place with God often held me together during these times when I wanted someone significant to share real intimacy with and still couldn't express into words what it was that I was seeking.

The authors of the book, **The Sacred Romance**,[iii] described what I was looking for in a way that resonated with me. The book is about the "attractiveness of God" and in 2020, I stumbled across their writings for the first time while doing some research. Best-selling author, John Eldredge and the late Brent Curtis authored **The Sacred Romance** and these gentlemen show how we long for intimacy, beauty, and adventure. When I heard how they described these three words in their book, I described it as 'the full package.' It is what I experience when I give myself completely to God and also what I want in a romantic relationship with a significant other.

Eldredge and Curtis talked about the external and internal persons that we as human being are. They explain, and I agree, how the external person is the person that everyone sees and knows us to be, while the internal person is the one that lives from within and is not easily seen, but very much longed for. The challenge is to allow the Holy Spirit to introduce you to that person inside of you that you very much want to be. One of the Scriptures the authors of **The Sacred Romance** use is found in **2 Corinthians 5:12**. This Scripture speaks of both the inner-person and the person seen by the outside world. It occurred to me as I read this Scripture and took in what the authors shared that this is more profound than I ever thought. We live in discord with ourselves because there are different facets of us that we never really get to know well. But the Holy Spirit's job, if we allow Him, is to show us who we really are and what we really want – both inside and out.

Even though God met me in my car years ago, I didn't know how to respond to that feeling I felt when He spoke to my heart. I didn't even really know how to share that testimony because nothing like that had ever happened to me. Going years without knowing how to respond to God as a Lover, or explain this phenomena, and stumbling across **The Sacred Romance** in 2020, I was thrilled to finally discover my full package. When it comes to life in general and life with another human being, I truly believe that the full package we look for in relationships consists of all three: intimacy, beauty, and adventure.

In every aspect of my being, I want to live a genuine authentic life. Regardless of whether I am at home alone or with the love of my life, whether I am at work, or in the supermarket, I am most fulfilled when I am able to just be genuinely me and accepted as such. The Holy Spirit shows us just who that person is and what that person really wants. That is one of His very important roles in our lives – if we will let Him.

DAY 7

Planning for the Best Dates Ever!

The Lord. The Lover. The Life Coach. SERIES™

DAY 7 – PLAN THE BEST DATES EVER!

What to Wear for Him

> **Psalm 143:10 KJV**
> ¹⁰ Teach me to do thy will; for thou art my God: thy spirit is good; lead me into the land of uprightness.

What do you wear for God on a date? Sounds like a strange question to ask. But I have found that when I treat Him like the King in my life – the Lover, He shows me that He is! Whatever I ask, whatever I desire in His pleasure is always mine. When I have not received what I expected from God, I have usually learned that there was something that I didn't know about it, but God did. My prayers began to change over time as God revealed more how to please Him.

Teach me to do thy will; for thou art my God: thy spirit is good; lead me into the land of uprightness. Let your abundant loving flow of power, blessing, honor, wisdom, strength, glory, and riches be mine and my offspring that you have given me forever. I want to be pregnant, not by an idol or the spirit of a thing, but by the one and only, sacred seed, which is Christ. I don't want to become pregnant by the thief. I don't want to be raped. I have a heavenly husband who loves me and he would not want to see me raped or violated. Therefore, I will wait for my King while He is at war. I will be His faith-filled Bride of Virtue. I will not take the bait of deception offered to my heart. I am Eve Reimagined. I am the one set free to love and be loved by God with all my heart, all my soul, and all my strength. Therefore, it will be well with me, for you have taught me to do thy will; you are my God: your spirit is good; you have led me into the land of uprightness, and have given me your love as a token of respect for your namesake. So that is what I will wear – the love you give.

Amen.

What to wear for him

How might your love & beliefs about interacting with God be affecting your love & beliefs about others?

What beliefs do you need to examine further about God

As Lord?

As Lover?

As Life Coach?

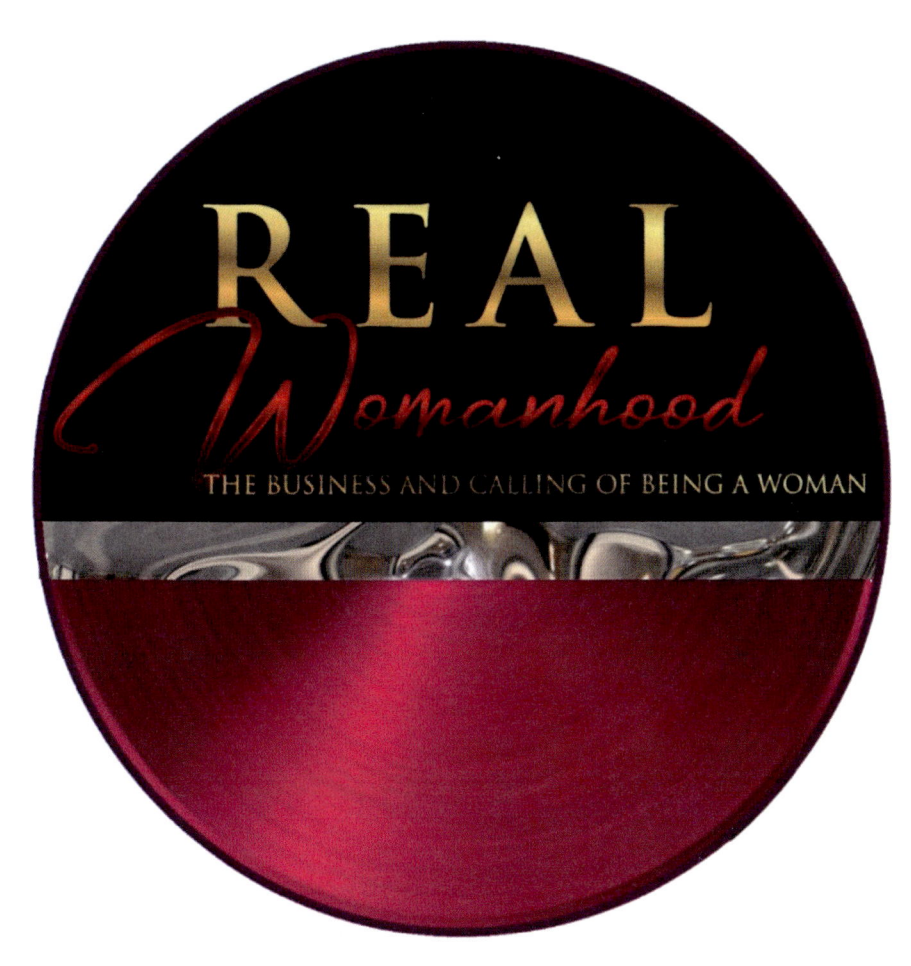

The Lord. The Lover. The Life Coach.
SERIES™

REAL Womanhood
THE BUSINESS AND CALLING OF BEING A WOMAN

Find other books by Dr. Merle Ray on:

- www.MyBestSeller.org
- www.RealWomanhood.com
- www.DrMerleRay.com
- Amazon and Barnes & Noble

Cited Sources:

_____

[i] CNBC. Why the coronavirus might change dating forever https://www.cnbc.com/2020/05/25/why-the-coronavirus-might-change-dating-forever.html last accessed 7-31-2020.

[ii] The phrase, "The Business and Calling of Being a Woman," is the intellectual property and curriculum developed by the author. **REALWomanhood: The Business and Calling of Being a Woman** logo and trademark are protected terms and may not be used without the written permission of Dr. Merle Ray, The Noble Groups.

[iii] The Sacred Romance: Drawing Closer to the Heart of God. Book by Brent Curtis and John Eldredge found on Amazon.com. Author's Website https://wildatheart.org/

Made in the USA
Middletown, DE
23 November 2022